The Eye in General Practice

Tenth Edition

R. D. Finlay
MA BM BCh (Oxon) FRCS FRCS (Edin) FRCOphth DO
Consultant Ophthalmic Surgeon, Royal United Hospital, Bath
Senior Examiner, Diploma Examination of the Royal College of
Ophthalmologists

P. A. G. Payne
MB BS (Lond) MRCS LRCP DO
General Practitioner
Hospital Practitioner, Bristol Eye Hospital
Tutor in Ophthalmology, University of Bristol

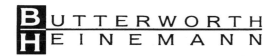

BUTTERWORTH
HEINEMANN

Butterworth-Heinemann
Linacre House, Jordan Hill, Oxford OX2 8DP
A division of Reed Educational and Professional Publishing Ltd

 A member of the Reed Elsevier plc group

OXFORD   BOSTON   JOHANNESBURG
MELBOURNE   NEW DELHI   SINGAPORE

First published by Longman Group Limited
First edition 1957   Sixth edition 1972
Second edition 1960   Seventh edition 1975
Third edition 1964   Eighth edition 1985
Fourth edition 1967   Ninth edition 1991
Fifth edition 1969   Tenth edition 1998

© Reed Education and Professional Publishing Ltd 1998

British Library Cataloguing in Publication Data
Finlay, R. D. (Robin Dundas)
   The eye in general practice. – 10th ed.
   1 Eye – Diseases
   I Title II Payne, P.A.G. III Jackson, C.R.S. (Charles Robert Sweeting)
   617.7

ISBN 0 7506 3691 2

Library of Congress Cataloguing in Publication Data
Finlay, R. D.
   The eye in general practice/R.D. Finlay, P.A.G. Payne. – 10th ed.
   p. cm.
   Rev. ed. of: The eye in general practice/C.R.S. Jackson, R.D. Finlay. 9th ed. 1991
   Includes bibliographical references and index.
   ISBN 0 7506 3691 2
   1 Eye–Diseases. 2 Ocular manifestations of general diseases. 3 Family medicine.
   I. Payne, P. A. G. II Jackson, C. R. S. (Charles Robert Sweeting) Eye in general
   practice. III Title.
   [DNLM: 1 Eye Diseases. 2 Family Practice. WW 140 F511e]
   RE65.J34
   617.7–dc21

Typesetting by David Gregson Associates, Beccles, Suffolk
Printed and bound in Spain

Contents

Preface

In preparing a 10th edition of *The Eye in General Practice*, the authors have principally in mind the needs of GPs, each of whom sees about three patients a week with an eye problem. Doctors working in Accident and Emergency Departments in both large and small hospitals, GP trainees and medical students are also regarded as potential users of the book.

The first edition was written in 1957 by Dr C. R. S. Jackson, who has since retired. The original preface set out his three objectives:

- To describe the common diseases of the eye
- To indicate danger signals and give help in deciding which cases should be referred immediately, which as routine referrals, and which can properly be managed in general practice
- To help the GP interpret reports sent back by hospital specialists and to discuss these with the patient, who may have returned from a hospital visit with the haziest of ideas about what occurred.

Optometrists now have very much wider clinical skills and expertise than was the case in 1957, and the GP is expected to evaluate their reports and explain them to the patient, as well as taking appropriate action.

Dr Jackson referred in his original preface to his own experience as a country GP before taking up ophthalmology. The present authors are a consultant ophthalmologist, who has vivid memories of deficiencies in knowledge and skills in ophthalmology while briefly working in general practice early in his career, and a GP who also practises part-time in a busy teaching eye hospital. He comes from a family of optometrists and so brings that additional perspective to his authorship.

The provision of clear and informative illustrations remains a high priority. Alterations to the ninth edition include a general update of all sections, including rapidly-changing fields such as refractive surgery and the management of infective diseases. There is a new chapter on the ocular associations of important systemic diseases.

The chapter on the interpretation of common presenting symptoms and signs has been modified. A description of the most readily-available type of slit-lamp microscope is included because these instruments are increasingly available to GPs, who may be encouraged to develop skill and confidence in their use.

Attending hospital eye clinics for a while, as assistant or observer, is probably the best way for a GP to supplement undergraduate and postgraduate teaching and to gain deeper insight into the everyday management of patients' eye problems. Sadly, there is insufficient time in a GP's training for this to be a routine for all. The authors hope that this book will earn a place on the shelves accessible to every GP and Accident and Emergency doctor, and also that it will be useful to medical students, ophthalmic nurses, optometrists and those helping people with impaired vision.

Acknowledgements

We are indebted to many colleagues for advice and, in particular for the present edition to Mr Rodney Grey, Mr Richard Harrad, Mr Bing Hoh, Dr Nicholas McLean, Mr Patrick Trevor-Roper, Dr Mala Viswalingham and Ms Caroline Dunford.

We acknowledge with thanks colleagues who have provided illustrations: Dr Tom Barrie of Glasgow, Mr David Boase of Portsmouth, Professor S. Darougar of London, Professor David Easty and Mr Christopher Dean Hart of Bristol, Mr Jack Kanski of Windsor, Mr Jonathan Luck, Dr Paul Lyons and Dr Michael Noakes of Bath, Dr Leslie Stokoe of Edinburgh and Mr John Strong of Swindon. Clement Clarke International Ltd and Keeler Ltd kindly allowed the reproduction of illustrations. Migraine art is reproduced by permission of the British Migraine Association and Boehringer Ingelheim.

Ms Gill Bennerson, of the Department of Medical Photography at Bristol Eye Hospital, was a great help, both in her enthusiasm and her support, as was Mr Simon Tutty of the Royal United Hospital, Bath. Miss Mollie Atkin, Valerie Walling and Margaret Nightingale kindly provided information about facilities for the visually impaired.

We are both enormously grateful for the help given by our secretaries, Mrs Marijane Inches and Miss Elinor Price.

R.D.F.
P.A.G.P.

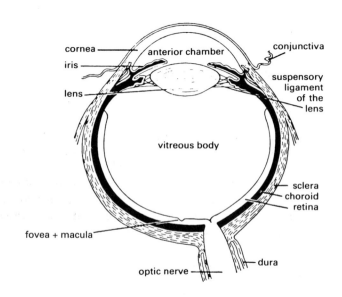

cornea

anterior chamber

conjunctiva

iris

suspensory
ligament
of the
lens

lens

vitreous body

sclera
choroid
retina

fovea + macula

dura

optic nerve

1
History and examination

Between 1% and 2% of patients attending GPs' surgeries do so on account of symptoms related to their eyes, so some attempt must be made to help in sorting out the various problems.

A GP might expect to see about 50 eye cases per 1000 patients on his/her list per year, most of which will be simple red eye conditions. The approximate incidence of other common eye diseases per 1000 patients on a GP's list is as follows:

Annually – 3–4 cataracts requiring
          referral for surgery
          1 diabetic retinopathy
          1 hypertensive retinopathy
Every 2 years – 1 retinal haemorrhage (excluding diabetes)
Every 3 years – a new case of glaucoma
Every 5 years – a retinal detachment

History

Problems may include pain, redness, watering, alteration in appearance, impaired or double vision. Commonly, blurred vision is reported by a patient as double – the distinction needs to be established. It must not be forgotten that some patients with eye or visual pathway disease may have no complaint.

There may be a history of previous similar episodes, of systemic illness, or of eye disease in the family; and the way in which symptoms first present may give clues. In particular, bilaterality or otherwise is important. A complaint of sudden visual loss may represent a sudden appreciation of a long-standing defect – as, for example, on happening to close or cover the 'good' eye.

Possible injury must not be overlooked, especially industrial injury through hammering, drilling, and so on. The nature and distribution of the pain may be important. The 'scratchy' pain of a superficial foreign body is quite distinct from the pain of deeper eye disease, which is often referred to brow or cheek, through the trigeminal nerve.

Essential equipment

An adequate initial examination of the eye can be made with simple apparatus. The following are the minimum requirements:

1. *Pen torch*. Held between finger and thumb, the disengaged fingers resting on the patient's face and helping to keep the eye open (Figure 1.1).

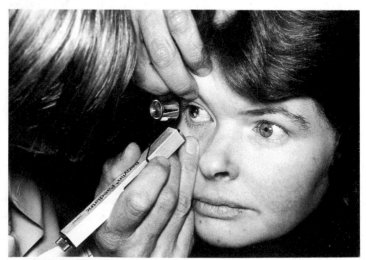

Fig. 1.1   Examination with torch and loupe

2. *Magnifier (x 8)*. For maximum field of view it must be held close to the examiner's eye. The standard auroscope, without the speculum, can be a useful tool in the surgery, especially if the room can be darkened.

3. *Fluorescein-impregnated paper strips* (Fluorets®) moistened with the tears in the lower part of the conjunctiva (Figure 1.2). (N.B. Never use fluorescein in bottles because of the danger of contamination, especially by *Pseudomonas*.) An alternative to fluorescein is rose bengal. A corneal epithelial defect will pick up the stain – green (fluorescein) or red (rose bengal).

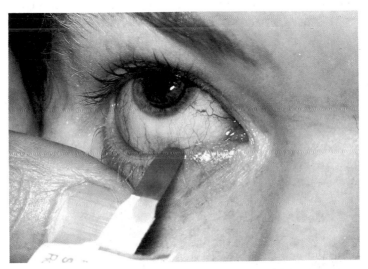

Fig. 1.2   Staining with fluorescein

4. *Quick-acting, short-lasting mydriatic*, to dilate the pupil if necessary. Useful drugs are cyclopentolate hydrochloride 0.5 or 1.0% (Mydrilate®), and tropicamide (Mydriacyl®) 0.5 or 1.0%. These are available in disposable, single-dose containers, as Minims®/Cyclopentolate and Minims®/Tropicamide respectively. Atropine should be avoided, its effects being unnecessarily prolonged. After the examination, a drop of pilocarpine 2% counteracts the effect of the mydriatic. (Mydriasis: dilatation of the pupil. Miosis: pupillary constriction.)

5. *Ophthalmoscope*. Several GP models are available, and are more useful if the battery is fresh and the bulb not blackened with age. A darkened room makes the examination easier. The ophthalmoscope remains the primary diagnostic tool in the GP's hands.

Essentially, it produces a bright beam of parallel light which can be focused by rotating different power lenses in front of the viewing hole. Its uses are not limited to retinal examination, and include:

a. General ocular examination. Using the right eye to examine the patient's right eye, and vice versa, the examiner should elevate the patient's upper lid with the thumb. Holding the ophthalmoscope about 2 cm from the patient's eye and with a +10 lens in the viewing hole, the cornea will be in focus (assuming both patient and examiner do not require spectacle corrections). By slowly reducing the power of the lens in the viewing hole, the examiner will be able to focus through the deeper media of the eye, until the retina comes into focus when a zero power lens is in position.

b. Retinal examination. It is sensible to develop a scheme of examination, to ensure that nothing is missed. Ideally one should start at the optic disc, which should be assessed for shape, colour and size of the cup, and then each of the four sectoral vessels should be followed to the periphery. The macula is best examined by asking the patient to look directly into the centre of the light of the ophthalmoscope.

c. Opacities within the eye. Corneal foreign bodies, lens opacities and vitreous opacities can all be viewed with the ophthalmoscope. The examiner should stand about half a metre away from the patient with a +3 lens in front of the viewing hole, and the beam of light should be directed through the patient's pupil to produce the red reflex. Any opacity will appear as a shadow within the pupil aperture. In the hands of an experienced examiner and by the use of parallax, the exact plane of the opacity can be assessed.

Dilating the pupils with a short-acting mydriatic as previously described is an essential part of ophthalmoscopy and makes fundus examination much easier. The commonly-held belief that acute angle-closure glaucoma may be precipitated is largely unfounded. Should it occur, it can be argued that it would almost certainly have occurred anyway, and it is preferable for it to do so in a controlled situation where the appropriate action can be taken swiftly. When examining a retina through an undilated pupil, it is often useful to use a small aperture of illumination, achieved by a control usually situated on the back of the ophthalmoscope.

6. *The slit-lamp microscope.* There are two basic components of the slit-lamp microscope – a source of light which produces an adjustable slit beam and a binocular microscope. The beam of light

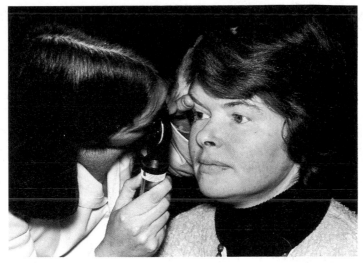

Fig. 1.3   Use of ophthalmoscope

can be shone into the media of the eye by swinging the mirror around in an arc of 180°. This allows the clear structures of the eye to be examined as a section in the slit light beam through the binocular microscope, thus providing a magnified stereoscopic image. This gives excellent views of the lids, conjuctiva, cornea, anterior chamber and lens. With the aid of diagnostic contact lenses, details of the drainage angle and canal of Schlemm and of the fundus can be examined by the experienced practitioner. Various filters can be added to the optical system – in particular, a blue filter is available for examining the cornea after it has been stained with fluorescein to demonstrate epithelial defects such as abrasions and ulcers. The slit beam of light can be reduced in size, and can be measured on a scale at the top of the instrument. This is particularly useful when the size of a lesion such as a hyphaema, corneal ulcer or iris melanoma needs monitoring. There are usually two magnification options on the microscope part of the slit-lamp, but the range can be increased by changing the removable eye pieces.

Simple scheme of examination

The first thing to do – and often overlooked – is to test the vision in each eye separately, with glasses if worn, for both distance and reading. (Some patients put on their reading glasses when invited to 'read' the distance test type!) Make sure that the eye not under test is adequately covered. Children, especially, are liable to 'peek'.

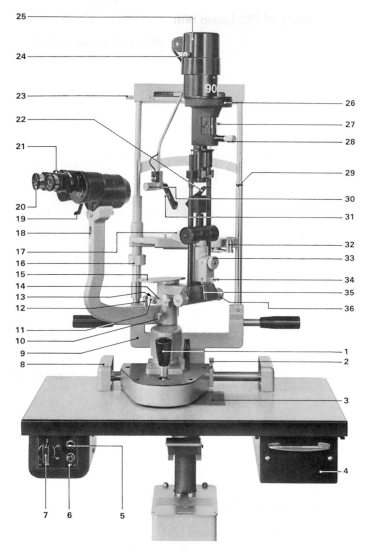

Fig. 1.4 Haag Streit 900 slit-lamp, model BM (Courtesy of Clement Clarke International Ltd)

The Snellen line labelled '6' (Fig. 1.5) can be read by the normal eye at 6m – hence 6/6. Diminishing ability is represented by 6/9, 6/12 and so on. Failure to achieve 6/60 is usually recorded as 'counting fingers' (CF), 'hand movements' (HM), 'perception of light' (PL) or 'no perception of light' (NPL).

Parts of Slit Lamp 900

1 Control lever for horizontal and vertical adjustment
2 Fixing screw for horizontal movements
3 Gliding plate
4 Accessory drawer
5 Pilot light
6 Fuse
7 Rotary switch
8 Rail covers
9 Headrest
10 Fixing screw for the microscope arm
11 2 knobs for coupling the microscope arm to the lamp arm
12 Roller for setting the angle between microscope and illumination
13 Index for reading angles
14 Scale for reading the angle between microscope and illumination
15 Guide plate for preset lens and applanation tonometer T 900.4.1
16 Level adjustment control for the chin rest
17 Chin rest

18 Fixing screw for the microscope
19 Lever for changing the objectives
20 Interchangeable eye-pieces
21 Knurled rings for setting the eye-pieces

22 Interchangeable illumination mirror
23 Knurled knob for lateral adjustment of the fixation light
24 Clamping nuts for the lamp housing
25 Cover for lamp housing
26 Scale for slit diaphragms
27 Lever for three filters
28 Control for rotation of slit, for varying the slit length and interposing the blue filter
29 Level marker
30 Fixation lamp
31 Handle for focusing the fixation target
32 Slide for preset lens
33 Centring screw
34 5° stops
35 Latch for the angle of inclination
36 Controls (2) for setting the slit width

A test card for near vision is useful, but a newspaper or telephone book will serve. For young children, and those who cannot read, some kind of illiterate test is needed. Letter matching tests such as the Sheridan Gardiner test (Fig. 1.6) or Stycar test are most frequently used. The child identifies a letter at 3 or 6m and matches it with one of a number of letters on a card held in his/her hand. Most children can manage this test at 3 years of age or older (see p. 187).

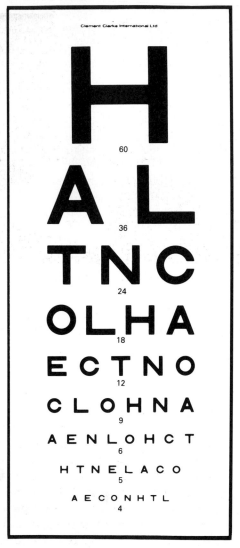

Fig. 1.5   Snellen test type (6m and 3m versions available)

If the patient has no glasses, or has left them at home, the 'pinhole' test may be of help. An eye in which defective vision is due to refractive changes or other 'anterior segment' problems will almost invariably have much improved vision when peering through a small hole punched in a piece of dark card. Plenty of light – and a steady hand – will be required, especially to examine the elderly,

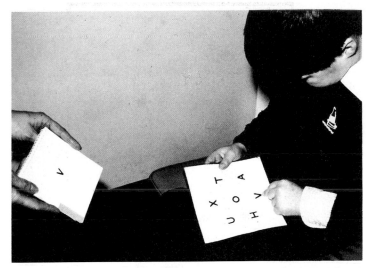

Fig. 1.6   Sheridan Gardiner test

but the satisfaction of demonstrating that the central retina is intact is significant, and it is reasonable to refer such patients to a local optometrist in the first instance.

Visual fields

The test of visual acuity takes account only of central vision. For completeness, a test of peripheral vision may be made by sitting in front of the patient and comparing the extent of his/her peripheral visual field with one's own, examining the eyes separately (Figure 1.7). At least, the ability to detect the movement of a hand in each of the four quadrants should be checked. This visual field test may reveal hemianopia from damage to the visual pathways, or field loss from glaucoma, both of which may exist in the presence of normal visual acuity, the patient being unaware of the defect.

A homonymous defect is most readily demonstrated by the examiner facing the patient and using both hands (Figure 1.8). Failure to see either hand indicates hemianopia; the defect is confirmed by moving the unseen hand across the midline, whereupon the patient is able to see both. This simple test should be repeated in the upper and lower quadrants. It may be helpful to ask the patient to count the examiner's fingers in different quadrants of the visual field where there is doubt about a defect.

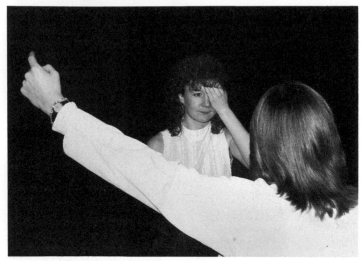

Fig. 1.7   Confrontation test for visual field

Eyelids

Symmetry on the two sides should be expected. Drooping or over-elevation of the upper lid may indicate ptosis or lid retraction, perhaps due to palsy of the oculomotor nerve or dysthyroid eye disease.

The skin around the eye is examined, and the normal position of the eyelashes noted. Inflammation of the lid margin may be noted, or swellings in the lid substance.

Surface of the eye

The patient must keep both eyes open. If this is difficult, a drop of short-acting local anaesthetic is invaluable – amethocaine hydro-chloride 1% or oxybuprocaine hydrochloride 0.4% (Minims® Benoxinate (Oxybuprocaine) Hydrochloride).

Redness most marked on the lining of the lids and around the periphery of the eye – conjunctivitis – should be differentiated from that which is duskier in colour and seen mostly around the margin of the cornea – ciliary congestion. The latter suggests disease of the cornea, iris, or deeper parts of the eye.

In the examination of the outer eye, the bright shiny surface of the cornea will be noted. Defects will be identified after the use of stain (see above).

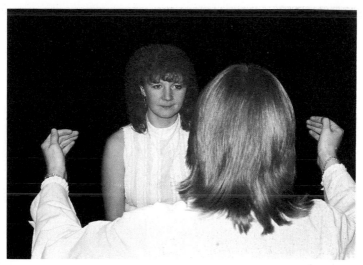

Fig. 1.8   Test for hemianopia

Pupils

The normal pupils are round, central and of equal size: they respond equally to light and to the need to accommodate. Examination involves four simple steps:

1. *Inspection.* Look for any irregularity of size, shape or position of either pupil.

2. *Light reaction.* With the fellow eye covered, shine the brightest light available (e.g. a pen torch, ophthalmoscope or desk light) directly into each eye in turn. A brisk, sustained contraction should be seen, the pupil dilating when the light is removed. The pupil of the eye not exposed to the light should constrict to the same extent – this is the consensual reaction.

3. *The swinging light test.* Illuminate first one eye and then the other. Each should show an equal and similarly-sustained pupil reaction. Dilatation of either pupil when illuminated indicates impaired conduction along the optic nerve on that side – a relative afferent pupillary defect. This is a simple and sensitive test of optic nerve function.

4. *Near response.* The patient is instructed to look into the distance and then at an object held close to his face: both pupils constrict, dilating again when distant gaze is resumed. The near response is invariably present if the light reflex is normal. Only in

the absence of a pupillary light reaction is a near response of relevance – 'light-near dissociation' (p. 170). Abnormalities of the pupil are discussed in Chapter 14.

Colour vision

Colour vision testing is sometimes of importance to the GP. There are two circumstances in which assessment can be of value:

1. *In optic nerve disorders* (Ch. 14) impaired colour recognition, especially of red, is an early finding. The colour may appear to be 'washed out' (desaturated), compared with its appearance when seen with the other eye. Red recognition is easily checked against that of the examiner by the confrontation test described for the visual field (Figure 1.7), using a red target. A red-topped pin or a small red plastic bottle top is satisfactory.

2. *Congenital colour blindness* occurs in various forms in about 8% of males and 0.4% of females, with sex-linked recessive inheritance. Detection of this defect is useful in routine visual screening, and patients sometimes ask to be tested. Specially designed tests are used for occupational testing, e.g. for airline and railway staff.

The *Ishihara* test is convenient for the GP. It consists of a book of coloured plates, each bearing a number that the patient has to identify.

Ocular movements

A complaint of double vision should be examined by moving an object in various directions, to find the direction in which double vision is present (see Figure 12.5).

Inner eye

Only practice can bring competence with the ophthalmoscope, and following a basic scheme of examination as described will ensure that nothing is missed. A complex diagnosis should not be expected, but it is essential that what is normal is recognized so that anything else can be referred appropriately.

2
Initial assessment

Symptoms have been discussed in Chapter 1. The remainder of the text is arranged on an anatomical basis, and the purpose of this chapter is to draw the two parts together, while reminding the reader that serious disease of the eye or visual pathway may exist in the absence of symptoms.

Presentation

Common presentations include:

1. Red eye
2. Pain
3. Visual loss – sudden or gradual
4. Distorted central vision
5. Haloes
6. Flashing lights
7. Spots before the eyes

1. *The red eye.* Most cases of 'red' eye can be dealt with at the first visit. Cases of doubt should be referred for initial diagnosis and treatment by an ophthalmologist, urgently if vision is affected (see Tables 2.1 and 2.2).

2. *Pain in the eye.* This may arise in the eye or be referred from elsewhere. Cases of persistent pain in the eye should be referred for urgent examination by an ophthalmologist (Table 2.3).

3. *Sudden loss of vision.* Visual loss may be total or partial, affecting only a sector of the visual field; it may be transient, or may persist. Unequivocally-diagnosed migraine (see p. 167) is the only condition for which urgent referral to an ophthalmologist is not mandatory. Patients over 60 years of age who have sudden

Table 2.1 The acute red eye

Diagnosis	History	Findings	Treatment
Subconjunctival haemorrhage (p. 40)	No pain	Redness confined beneath conjunctiva	None, if trauma excluded
Conjunctivitis (p. 42)	Painless or mild discomfort	Bulbar and palpebral conjunctiva affected Sticky eye – difficulty opening on waking	Antibiotic drops or ointment if infective Steroid drops if acute allergic reaction
Episcleritis (p. 51)	Painless or mild discomfort	Only bulbar conjunctiva affected Nodular or diffuse No discharge	Steroid or non-steroidal anti-inflammatory drops or ointment
Keratitis (p. 59)	Moderate pain and photophobia: vision may be affected	Loss of corneal clarity Cornea stains with fluorescein Engorged vessels radiating from limbus (ciliary congestion)	Refer
Iritis (p. 70)	Moderate pain and photophobia: vision may be affected	Ciliary congestion Tarsal conjunctiva not affected Small ± distorted pupil	Refer
Scleritis (p. 52)	Deep-seated pain	Deep, dusky redness ± swelling of sclera Frequently associated with connective tissue disorder	Refer
Acute angle-closure glaucoma (p. 145)	Severe pain ± vomiting Marked visual impairment Haloes around lights	Corneal haze (oedema) Oval, semidilated pupil Eye stony-hard to palpation/tonometry	Refer urgently

N.B. Always test the visual acuity.

Table 2.2 Chronic red, sore, irritable eyes: principal causes

Diagnosis	History	Findings	Management
Allergic conjunctivitis (p. 47)	Allergy/atopy Itching	Papillae on palpebral conjunctiva Excoriation of eyelid skin	Topical mast cell stabilizer (e.g. sodium cromoglycate) Steroid drops (short course, <4 weeks) Oral antihistamine Identify cause(s) if possible
Blepharitis –Anterior/seborrhoeic (p. 22)	Crusty/inflamed lid margins Tarsal cysts	Anterior lid margins involved – scales/ulceration Scalp seborrhoea	Lid scrubs Antibiotic drops Steroid drops (short course only)
–Posterior (p. 23)		Posterior lid margins affected; inflamed Meibomian orifices along centre of lid margin ± tarsal cysts ± rosacea	Lid soaking with warm compresses Meibomian gland expression Topical antibiotics ± oral tetracycline
Chronic conjunctivitis –Conjunctivitis medicamentosa (pp 126)	Persistent red eye ± history of topical medication	Often minimal signs	Stop all medication and review Refer if diagnosis in doubt
–Chlamydial conjunctivitis (p. 44)	May be unilateral Sexually-active individual	Follicles in lower fornix	Refer
–Molluscum contagiosum (p. 26)	Unilateral	Typical umbilicated lesion on adjacent lid	Refer or remove lesion
Dry eye (p. 36)	Symptoms variable, worse in evenings, indoors or in heated car ± dry mouth ± collagen disorder	Rose bengal staining of cornea/conjunctiva	Tear supplements Refer difficult cases
Others –Eyelid malpositions (p. 27)		Ectropion/entropion	Refer
–Lagophthalmos (p. 65)	Symptoms worse on waking	Incomplete lid closure ± associated dry eye	Ocular lubricants on retiring at night
–Trichiasis (p. 27)		Inturning eyelashes	Refer
–Dermatoses (p. 30)	Atopy Drug/cosmetic application	Local skin irritation Oedema and redness	Identify cause ?Refer to dermatologist or eye clinic

N.B. Always test the visual acuity.

Table 2.3   Pain attributed to the eye

	Condition	Features

Major painful eye disorders	Cornea
	  Keratitis (p. 59)
	  Abrasion (p. 56) ·
	  Foreign body (p. 58)
		Ciliary congestion; fluorescein staining.

	Iritis (p. 70)	Ciliary congestion; small, irregular pupil; vision may be impaired.
	Scleritis (p. 52)	Usually associated systemic disorder.
	Acute glaucoma (p. 145)	Corneal oedema; fixed, semidilated pupil; shallow anterior chamber; hard eye; may be vomiting.

Eye disorders causing discomfort	Lids
	  Entropion (p. 28)
	  Trichiasis (p. 27)
		Malpositioned or loose lashes.

	Conjunctiva
	  Conjunctivitis (p. 42)
	  Dry eye (p. 36)
		Palpebral and bulbar conjunctiva inflamed; discharge.
		Rose bengal punctate staining; Schirmer's test.

	Episcleritis (p. 51)	Nodular or diffuse.
	Optic neuritis (p. 162)	Vision impaired; colour desaturation; afferent pupillary defect; discomfort on palpating globe; may be disc swelling.

Pain referred to the eye	Trigeminal nerve
	  Herpes zoster
	    ophthalmicus (p. 61)
	  Trigeminal neuralgia
		Rash.
		
		Lancinating pain; trigger zone.

	Sinusitis	Tender on pressure over sinus; radiograph.
	Scalp (p. 160) Giant cell arteritis	Tenderness; raised ESR/plasma viscosity; may lead to sudden visual loss (ischaemic optic neuropathy).
	Neck Tension headache	Continuous, symmetrical pain; not associated with visual or gastrointestinal symptoms.

	Intracranial
	  Migraine (p. 167)
	
	  Migrainous neuralgia
		Aura; distribution; duration; gastrointestinal symptoms.
		'Cluster' incidence; unilateral; associated lacrimal and nasal discharge.

	Raised intracranial
	    pressure (p. 164)
	
	  Intracranial aneurysm
		Papilloedema; nausea/vomiting; headache worse in morning and on coughing/straining.
		Associated cranial nerve lesion.

	Refractive error (p. 123)	Symptoms suggest eye-strain; refer for refraction in first instance.
	Ocular muscle imbalance (p. 139)	

visual loss must have an ESR or plasma viscosity check immediately, to detect asymptomatic giant cell arteritis. Missing this diagnosis may result in visual loss in the second eye and total blindness which could have been prevented. The principal causes of sudden loss of vision are given in Table 2.4.

Table 2.4   Sudden loss of vision

Site	Cause	Features
Vitreous	Massive vitreous haemorrhage (p. 93)	Loss of red reflex on fundus examination. *Red reflex*
Retina	Retinal arterial occlusion (p. 89)	Branch – partial loss of vision. Central – total loss of vision and of direct pupillary reaction. *fundoscopy*
	Central retinal vein occlusion (p. 91)	Extensive haemorrhage in fundus.
	Amaurosis fugax (p. 91)	'Curtain' over vision, usually recovering in minutes. Embolus may be visible in retinal arteriole. Carotid bruit may be present. *Auscultate carotids c murmurs*
	Retinal detachment involving macula (p. 104)	Flashing lights, 'floaters', and visual field loss spreading centrally.
Optic nerve	Ischaemic optic neuropathy (p. 160)	Afferent pupillary defect, disc swelling a. 'Anterior ischaemic' – usually partial visual loss. b. Giant cell arteritis – ESR/viscosity raised. *pupillary reflex + palpate temporal area.*
	Optic neuritis (p. 162)	Age group 20–45 years. Central field defect – peripheral field intact. Eye tender on palpation and on looking sideways. Impaired direct pupillary light reaction (p. 11). Spontaneous recovery usual in 2–4 weeks. *palpate eye.*
Visual pathway	Stroke (p. 167)	Homonymous hemianopia (the patient may think it unilateral). Total visual loss if previous hemianopia unrecognized, or cortical blindness. Normal pupil reactions.
	Migraine (p. 167)	Characteristic aura and recovery. Scintillating scotoma; flashing lights. Gastrointestinal symptoms. Recovery almost invariable.
Acute glaucoma (p. 145)		Pain ± vomiting. Red eye. Corneal oedema. Semidilated pupil. Eye stony-hard.
Toxic reactions (p. 163)		Quinine or methyl alcohol poisoning.

N.B. Apparently sudden loss of vision may be due to the discovery of a pre-existing defect or may be functional. Referral is always justified.

4. *Gradual loss of vision.* The commonest causes are given in Table 2.5.

Table 2.5   Gradual loss of vision

	Cause	Features
Lens	Cataract (p. 76)	Increased myopia or blurring.
Retina	Macular degeneration (p. 94)	Straight lines appear distorted. Peripheral field unaffected.
	Retinal vein occlusion (p. 91)	Typical retinal haemorrhages.
	Retinal detachment (p. 104)	Flashing lights and 'floaters' Visual field loss spreading centrally.
Optic nerve nerve	Chronic glaucoma (p. 147)	Usually so gradual as to pass unnoticed. Optic disc cupping, raised intraocular pressure and field loss.
	Toxic optic neuropathy	Heavy smoking and/or alcohol intake. Peripheral field intact.
Visual pathway	Compressive lesions of visual pathway.	Must be excluded if no other cause found. Temporal field defect usual. CT scan required.

5. *Distorted central vision* may be caused by
   a. Retinal detachment beginning to involve macula (p. 104)
   b. Macular degeneration of any type (p. 94)
   c. Macular haemorrhage.
Pupillary light reaction is normal. Dilatation of the pupil is essential for satisfactory examination.

6. *Haloes* round lights may be due to
   a. Raised intraocular pressure in angle-closure glaucoma (p. 145)
   b. Corneal disease.
   c. Lens opacities.
Always refer the patient for investigation, to exclude angle-closure glaucoma.

7. *Flashing lights* before one or both eyes – the patient may not be sure which – may be due to
   a. Teichopsia (scintillating scotoma) of migraine (Figure 14.9)
   b. Retinal tear (p. 104)
   c. Retinal detachment (p. 104)
   d. Vitreous detachment (p. 86).

Unless the history of migraine is certain, refer the patient for detailed retinal examination.

8. *Spots before the eyes* may be caused by
   a. Vitreous haemorrhage
   b. Uveitis with vitreous opacities (p. 69)
   c. Retinal tear with operculum lying in the vitreous (p. 104)
   d. Posterior vitreous detachment occurring suddenly
   e. 'Innocent' degenerative changes in the vitreous (p. 86).

This list contains enough vision-threatening conditions to justify referral of the patient if the GP is not entirely satisfied that the condition is due to innocent vitreous opacities. Flashing lights and spots before the eyes are a particularly dangerous combination, referral of the patient being essential.

Referrals

Except in an emergency, when contact is likely to be made by telephone, the majority of patients referred to the ophthalmologist will have been examined initially by an optometrist. The optometrist will send a letter or a completed proforma to the GP. This report contains details of the findings, and it should be sent, complete, to the ophthalmologist with the referral letter.

The optometrist's report will record the visual acuity, the spectacle correction and other findings. If this information is available to the ophthalmologist, repetition of some tests will be avoided and the point of the referral will not be missed. Also of importance are details of the patient's general state of health, with information about relevant past illnesses and family history. These are especially helpful in the case of elderly patients who may not be good at recalling information. A recent blood pressure reading and the result of a urine test for glucose will also be appreciated by the ophthalmologist, together with a list of any drugs that the patient is currently taking.

The degree of urgency with which a patient should be seen by the ophthalmologist can form the basis for grouping the reasons for referral, as follows:

1. *Emergency* cases should be sent directly to the Accident and Emergency Department. They include:
   perforating injury, suspected or known intraocular foreign body, suspected or known chemical burns
   sudden loss of vision
   hypopyon (p. 59)
   acute angle-closure glaucoma.

2. *Urgent* cases should be seen within 24 hours. They may involve:
   retinal detachment
   orbital fracture
   hyphaema or vitreous haemorrhage
   ocular inflammation of sudden onset, e.g. iritis or ophthalmic herpes zoster
   corneal foreign bodies or abrasions
   corneal ulcer
   sudden onset of diplopia or squint associated with pain.

3. *Moderately urgent* cases should be seen within 1–2 weeks, and may involve:
   'floaters'
   flashing lights without a field detect
   open-angle glaucoma with pressure >35 mmHg.

4. *Routine* cases may involve:
   chalazion/stye/cysts
   ptosis
   headaches and migraine
   gradual loss of vision
   chronic open-angle glaucoma (unless pressure >35 mmHg)
   chronic red eye conditions
   painless diplopia or squint.

3
The eyelids

Anatomy

The skin of the lid is thin and without subcutaneous fat. Inflammation or trauma leads to much swelling.

The margin of the upper lid normally crosses the upper third of the cornea, and the lower lid margin lies at the lower limbus (junction of cornea and sclera). Exposure of sclera below the cornea is one of the first signs of proptosis.

The tarsal or Meibomian glands lie in the substance of the lid and discharge at the lid margin.

In front, the lids have two or three rows of lashes, while the inner end of each lid carries the lacrimal punctum, the upper end of the lacrimal drainage apparatus, which is invisible unless the lid is everted.

The orbicularis muscle, supplied by the facial nerve, encircles the orbit and is responsible for blinking and for forced protective closure of the eye. The levator of the upper lid is supplied by the third cranial nerve.

Wounds of the lids

These injuries require special attention because they may accompany an injury to the eyeball. Lid wounds are best treated in a specialist unit, as the distortion resulting from incorrect alignment may lead to unsightly notching of the lid margin, distortion of the lashes or interference with lacrimal drainage.

Destructive injuries of the lids may expose the cornea, which must on no account be allowed to become dry. Pending repair, the cornea should be protected by the use of plenty of antibiotic ointment and a pad.

Inflammation of the lids

Blepharitis

Blepharitis (inflammation of the lid margins) is of two types: anterior and posterior.

Anterior (seborrhoeic) blepharitis (Figure 3.1a)

This gives rise to chronically irritable eyes; the lid margins are reddened and conjunctivitis is present. Crusts are seen at the roots of the lashes. Seborrhoea capitis is a common association.

Treatment is tedious. The patient is instructed to apply warm compresses to the lids for a few minutes several times a day, and then to scrub the lid margins with a cotton bud moistened in a solution of a few drops of baby shampoo in half a cupful of warm, boiled water. A dilute solution of bicarbonate of soda is an alternative to shampoo. The purpose of this scrubbing is to remove the crusts from the bases of the lashes. Then, in exacerbations, antibiotic ointment may be rubbed into the lid margin or drops instilled. The addition of a topical steroid for not more than 4 weeks at a time is useful in severe cases. Regular hair washing with a medicated shampoo and scrupulous washing of the face help to control chronic seborrhoea.

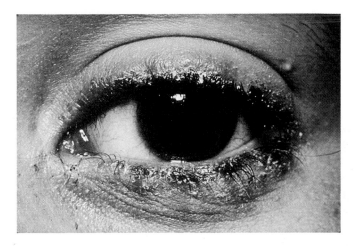

Fig. 3.1a   Anterior blepharitis, seborrhoeic type: note crusting of eyelashes

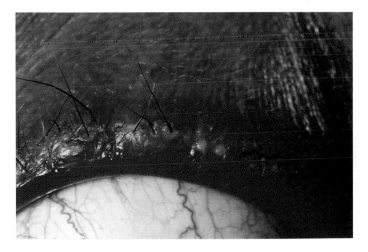

Fig. 3.1b   Anterior blepharitis: staphylococcal infection of follicles (folliculitis) and loss of lashes

Posterior blepharitis (see Figure 6.6, p. 64)

The characteristic finding is pouting and excessive discharge from the Meibomian gland openings, which are situated in the gray line on the lid margin. The entire lid margin is hyperaemic and there may be chalazia (see below).

Treatment involves moistening and warming the lids with a flannel soaked in hot water, and then massaging the lid with a cotton bud using a stroking action, upwards on the lower lids and downwards on the upper lids, to express retained Meibomian secretions.

Posterior blepharitis is commonly associated with rosacea, and when active a 2-month course of tetracycline 250 mg b.d. taken between meals is helpful in addition to lid cleansing. Rosacea may be associated with serious eye complications and persistent cases should be referred.

Hordeolum (stye)

This is an abscess in one of the glands related to a lash follicle. Pointing occurs in the line of the lashes, distinguishing this condition from the chalazion.

Treat by hot bathing and antibiotic ointment. A thermos flask filled with boiling water, held under the eye, is an easy way to apply steam to the eye.

Swellings of the lids

Benign

Chalazion (Meibomian, or tarsal, cyst) (Figure 3.2)

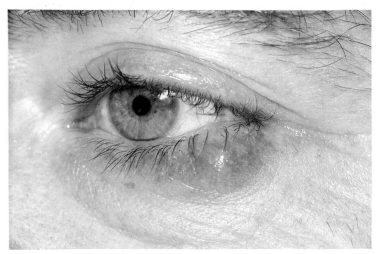

Fig. 3.2   Chalazion (tarsal cyst)

This is a chronic swelling in the substance of the lid, painless unless abscess formation occurs. Characteristically, it is centred some distance from the lid margin and thus distinguished from a stye. Chalazia are often multiple and repeated, and are common in association with rosacea.

Treatment consists of incision and curettage. This is an outpatient procedure which a GP may wish to undertake. The equipment required is: *

Chalazion clamp
Chalazion curette
Fine scissors and forceps
Scalpel (No. 11 or 15 blade)
Anaesthetic drops (amethocaine hydrochloride 1% or oxybuprocaine hydrochloride 0.4%)
Local anaesthetic for injection
Antibiotic ointment
Eyepad and swabs.

Technique: Anaesthetize the conjunctiva with drops. Inject 1–2 ml of 1–2% lignocaine around the swelling, through the skin surface. Apply the clamp so that the cyst protrudes through the ring on the conjunctival side. Open the cyst by means of a vertical incision and curette out the (usually gelatinous) contents. It may be necessary to excise granulation tissue with scissors and forceps. Instil antibiotic ointment and apply a firm pad over the closed eye. Local pressure should be maintained for 10 min. or so. The pad can then usually be discarded. The eye should be bathed, and antibiotic ointment instilled, twice daily for about 3 days.

Other cysts

Sebaceous cysts and molluscum contagiosum (Figure 3.3) need surgical evacuation.

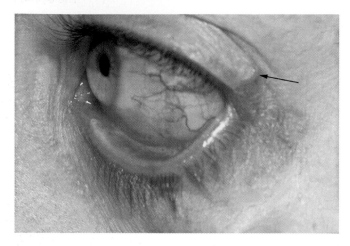

Fig. 3.3   Molluscum contagiosum: note lesion on upper lid and mild conjunctivitis

Xanthelasma (Figure 3.4)

Common in the elderly and in diabetics, these flat creamy plaques may be removed on cosmetic grounds. They may signify hyperlipidaemia.

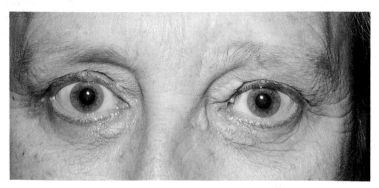

Fig. 3.4   Xanthelasma

Malignant

Basal-cell carcinoma (rodent ulcer) (Figure 3.5)

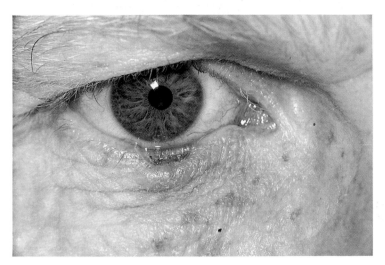

Fig. 3.5   Basal cell carcinoma (rodent ulcer) of lower lid: note potential contusion with a tarsal cyst

This has characteristic rolled edges, and is typically seen in Europeans who have been exposed over many years to bright sunlight. It is the commonest malignancy in the eyelid, slow-growing and only locally invasive. If untreated, it leads to considerable loss of tissue.

Treatment is by either local excision with at least 2 mm of surrounding tissue, radiotherapy or cryotherapy, depending on the size and site of the lesion.

Squamous carcinoma (epithelioma)

This requires wide excision, with diagnostic biopsy.

Malpositions

Trichiasis

Trichiasis is the turning inwards of the eyelashes, and may result from wounds or inflammation. The abnormal lashes rub against the globe, with irritation, watering and potential damage to the cornea.

Treatment is difficult; simple epilation may suffice, or the offending lashes can be eliminated by electrolysis or cryotherapy. Difficult cases should be referred.

Entropion (Figure 3.6)

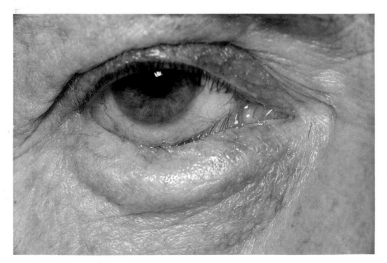

Fig. 3.6   Entropion

This is a backward rolling of the lid edge, the lashes actually disappearing from view, and occurs mostly in the elderly (senile spastic entropion). It may occur spontaneously or follow irritation. If intermittent, entropion may be induced by asking the patient to close the eye forcibly. Temporary relief can be obtained by the use of a strip of plaster between the lid and the cheek, but recurrent or persistent entropion needs surgery and must therefore be referred.

Ectropion (Figure 3.7)

The edge of the lower lid may fall away from the eye as a result of wounds or inflammation, but most commonly in facial palsy or senile loss of tone in the facial muscles. The principal complaint will be of watering. Later, there will be conjunctivitis and increased discharge.

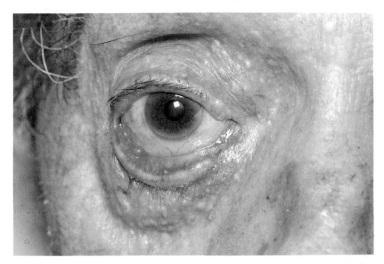

Fig. 3.7 Ectropion: in mild cases, only the medial part of the lid is affected

Treatment is surgical, but the patient should be taught not to make the condition worse by wiping his eyes downwards. He should wipe them upwards and medially towards the nose.

Ptosis (Figure 3.8)

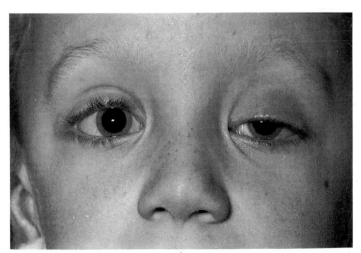

Fig. 3.8 Congenital ptosis - 3rd cr - n

Ptosis, or drooping of the upper lid, occurs in palsy of the third cranial nerve and may result from a multitude of neurological conditions. It is a diagnostic sign of myasthenia gravis, and may be induced or made worse by asking the patient to gaze steadily at a finger held in front of his face and above the horizontal plane.

Of greater importance from the ophthalmic point of view is congenital ptosis – unilateral or bilateral, complete or partial. It is often associated with limited elevation of the affected eye, due to weakness of the superior rectus muscle. It is impossible to mistake a child suffering from bilateral congenital ptosis, with the characteristic 'head back' attitude in his/her attempt to see through the reduced palpebral aperture.

Treatment is surgical, and the timing of the operation depends on the child's age and whether or not there is a risk of the eye becoming amblyopic ('lazy') due to stimulus deprivation resulting from the pupil being covered by the lid.

Congenital ptosis is sometimes associated with epicanthus (Figure 12.2, p. 136), a prominent fold of skin overlying the inner corner of the eye. This usually improves with age but may require complex surgery.

Senile ptosis is common, and usually involves disinsertion of the levator muscle complex from the tarsal plate. It may follow other ocular surgery.

A minor degree of ptosis constitutes part of Horner's syndrome (see p. 169).

Dermatoses

Itching and burning eyelids, accompanied by redness, oedema, scaling and weeping often present a diagnostic problem for GP, ophthalmologist and dermatologist alike. There are two main groups of dermatoses:

Allergic/irritant contact dermatitis (Figure 3.9)

The administration of drugs, particularly atropine and topical antibiotics such as neomycin, is frequently the cause of redness and swelling of the eyelids.

Removal of the cause effects a cure, but more rapid symptomatic relief may be obtained in severe cases by the use of 1% hydrocortisone cream three or four times per 24 hours.

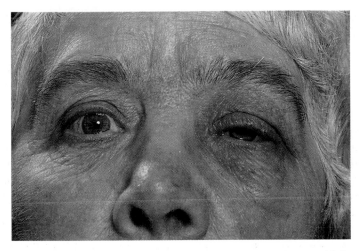

Fig. 3.9   Allergic contact dermatitis, due to antibiotic/steroid drops after cataract surgery to left eye

Irritant contact dermatitis, when there is direct irritation rather than a type IV hypersensitivity reaction, is generally less severe.

Atopic dermatitis

Patients with this condition usually have a personal and family history of eczema, asthma or hay fever. Ectropion may occur, and secondary infection leads to loss of lashes. Conjunctival and corneal involvement are common (see pp. 42, 48).

Management can be difficult, involving cold water compresses, simple ointments, oral antihistamines and topical steroids. Associated infection requires topical antibiotics. Systemic steroids are best avoided.

Facial palsy

Idiopathic facial palsy (Bell's palsy) may lead to exposure keratitis. In the early stage, this is best prevented by applying ointment, usually containing an antibiotic such as chloramphenicol or an ocular lubricant, liberally to the eye at night. If the eye becomes inflamed or corneal damage is demonstrated, the patient should be referred. Joining the lids by lateral tarsorrhaphy protects the cornea.

Involuntary movements

Recognized as an everyday occurrence in response to injury or threat of injury, forcible closure of the eye is so common as to appear scarcely worthy of mention. When, however, blepharospasm occurs without warning and in the presence of a normal eye, it may become a matter of serious concern.

A degree of fibrillary twitching in one or more of the facial muscles is probably universal, and may amount to no more than a mild embarrassment, particularly when unilateral. Bilateral involuntary closure of the eyes, with temporary total blindness as a result, requires treatment. Selective denervation of the orbicularis muscle is the treatment of choice, most readily achieved by the injection of minute quantities of botulinum toxin into the muscle. The injection may be expected to give relief for up to 6 months, and can be repeated.

Blepharoplasty

This is a term used to describe a number of cosmetic surgical procedures to correct laxity of the eyelid skin. Complications may occur and the surgeon has an obligation to ensure that eye and adnexal disorders are evaluated before undertaking treatment.

4
The lacrimal system

Anatomy and physiology
The watery eye
  – Epiphora from overproduction of tears
  – Epiphora from failure of outflow
The dry eye

Anatomy and physiology (Figure 4.1)

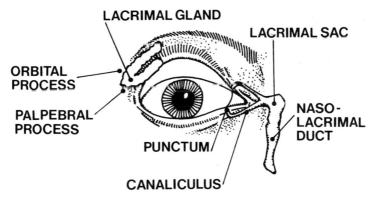

Fig. 4.1   The lacrimal apparatus

The lacrimal gland lies in the upper outer corner of the orbit and drains into the conjunctival sac. The tears are carried by movements of the lids to the inner corner of the eye. On each lid, at the inner end, is a minute lacrimal punctum, invisible until the lid is everted. Both the upper and lower canaliculi carry the tears to the lacrimal sac, from which the nasolacrimal duct drains to the inferior meatus of the nose.

The conjunctiva is normally moistened by mucous and accessory lacrimal glands, the lacrimal gland providing extra lubrication when needed.

The watery eye

Abnormal watering (epiphora) is caused by overproduction of tears or interference with outflow. The symptomatic relief of epiphora may be achieved by drops containing zinc sulphate 0.25%, used on a p.r.n. basis.

Epiphora from overproduction of tears

This may be due to:

1. Irritation of conjunctiva or cornea, as by a conjunctival or corneal foreign body, or conjunctivitis.
2. Irritation of the fifth cranial nerve (reflex epiphora).
3. Exposure to bright light (reflex epiphora).

Epiphora from failure of outflow

The causes may be as follows:

1. Malposition of the punctum, which then fails to pick up the tears.
2. Occasionally a loose lash gets washed into the punctum, giving a characteristic patch of redness where it rubs against the conjunctiva. Removal of the lash produces a gratifyingly rapid cure.
3. Obstruction in the canaliculus. Canalicular blockage is a rare cause of epiphora: it sometimes follows trauma.
4. Obstruction in the nasolacrimal duct:
    a. *In infancy.* The commonest cause of unilateral conjunctivitis in a baby is an obstructed nasolacrimal duct; such conjunctivitis is often recurrent. The nasolacrimal apparatus develops from a solid cord of ectodermal cells folded into the face along the groove between the frontonasal and maxillary processes. Subsequent canalization leads to the formation of the lacrimal sac and nasolacrimal duct. In some cases, canalization is incomplete.

    There is no abnormality during the first weeks of life, and then the eye becomes watery and tends to be sticky. Finger pressure over the lacrimal sac may produce a reflux of mucoid material from the punctum. Conservative treatment is worthwhile for a few weeks.

The child's mother is instructed to keep the sac empty by finger pressure several times a day, and to use antibiotic drops. Many cases resolve spontaneously, but failure to do so is an indication for probing of the duct – an outpatient procedure carried out under general anaesthetic, but not normally before the child is 1 year old as the nasolacrimal duct will often canalize spontaneously within the first 12 months of life.

b. *In the adult.* Chronic obstruction of the nasolacrimal duct is often due to dacryocystitis, which is more common in women than in men, and occurs usually after the menopause. Chronic dacryocystitis leads to constant watering of the eye and may be associated with the development of a mucocele from which mucopus can be expressed by finger pressure over the lacrimal sac. Not only is the obstructed duct liable to acute inflammation, it is also a reservoir from which infected material constantly enters the conjunctival sac. This means that any injury to the eye is liable to become infected, and any operation is similarly at risk. Any obstruction to the lacrimal system can be clearly seen on x-ray film, by means of a dacryocystogram.

It is a relatively simple procedure to syringe the nasolacrimal duct to confirm obstruction, and this can easily be carried out in general practice if the appropriate equipment is available. The conjunctival sac is anaesthetized with a drop of amethocaine hydrochloride 1% or oxybuprocaine hydrochloride 0.4%. The lower punctum is identified and a 25-gauge disposable lacrimal cannula, attached to a 2 ml syringe containing normal saline, is inserted into the lower canaliculus. Saline is then injected into the duct, which if obstructed will cause regurgitation through either the lower or upper punctum, depending on the exact site of the obstruction. If the duct is patent, the patient will be able to feel the saline drain into the throat.

In most cases the treatment of dacryocystitis is by the creation of a new channel to the nose. Dacryocystorhinostomy (DCR) consists of making an anastomosis between the lacrimal and nasal mucous membranes. The tears can then enter the nose, bypassing the obstructed nasolacrimal duct.

The dry eye

Inadequate tear production is an important cause of ocular discomfort, and contributes to many cases of failure to tolerate contact lenses. Tear secretion naturally decreases with advancing age. The patient with inadequate tear production complains of vague irritation and attacks of redness of the eyes. The symptoms are variable, and tend to be worst in centrally-heated buildings, in cars with the heater blowing hot air, or in any situation which increases the spontaneous drying of the eyes. Inadequate tear production is more common in post-menopausal women, and should be investigated in the young.

Patients with collagen disorders, particularly rheumatoid arthritis, are prone to a more severe form of keratoconjunctivitis sicca, characterized by diminished tear and salivary secretion, with dryness of the cornea and formation of filaments on its surface (this combination of features being known as Sjögren's syndrome). The symptoms are discomfort and, sometimes, mucoid discharge, occasionally progressing to frank corneal ulceration with severe pain.

Tear production is assessed by Schirmer's test (Figure 4.2). The conjunctiva is anaesthetized with a local anaesthetic drop. A strip of filter paper 5 mm wide is placed over the margin of the lower lid and removed after 5 minutes. The length of the strip wetted is measured: 15 mm or more represents normal tear production.

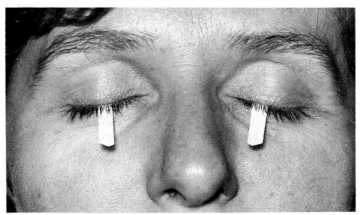

Fig. 4.2   Schirmer's test

Staining the cornea and conjunctiva with rose bengal (obtainable in solution as Minims® Rose Bengal) after the instillation of a drop of topical anaesthetic is another method of assessing the adequacy of tear secretion. Dry eyes show multiple small red dots on the cornea and conjunctiva, representing punctate epithelial defects, when examined under magnification. Mucous filaments may be seen adhering to the cornea (filamentary keratitis) (Figures 4.3a and 4.3b).

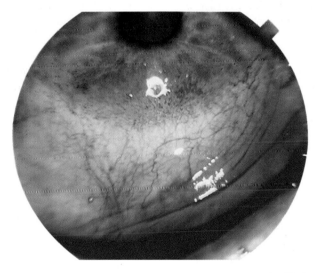

Fig. 4.3a   Dry eye: punctate staining with rose bengal of inferior cornea and conjunctiva

Although defective tear production cannot be cured, symptomatic relief can be obtained by the use of artificial tear supplements. Frequency of use varies with the severity of symptoms, and may range from every 30 minutes to once or twice a day. There are numerous commercially-available brands of tear supplements, most in drop form and containing preservative. Some are available in 'single dose' units and are preservative-free. Viscotears liquid gel® and Lacri-lube® are dispensed from tubes and may be easier to instil by some patients. Patients may be advised to try several different preparations, and to persist with that which is most acceptable. It should be remembered that it is often cheaper to buy artificial tears over the counter than by prescription.

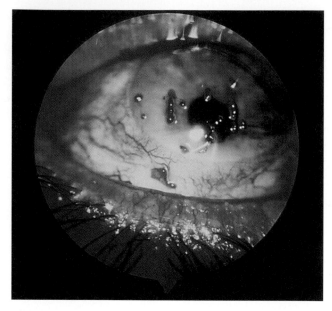

Fig. 4.3b   Dry eye: mucous filaments stained with rose bengal

Patients whose dry eyes cause distress in spite of the use of artificial tears should be referred for assessment by an ophthalmologist. Measures to conserve tears, such as surgical occlusion of the lacrimal puncta with cautery, may be helpful. Mucolytic drops such as acetylcysteine 5% (Ilube®) may also be recommended.

5
Conjunctiva and sclera

Anatomy

The conjunctiva covers the anterior part of the eye and lines the lids. Its numerous glands moisten the surface. Lubrication is also provided by the lacrimal gland. Tears contain lysozyme, which inhibits the growth of organisms.

Deep to the conjunctiva is the sclera; the episclera is the layer in between.

Conjunctiva

Lacerations

Conjunctival wounds need to be treated with respect, for there may be a concealed injury to the eye. Visual acuity must be checked. Conjunctival tissue heals rapidly if the wound edges are in apposition. Gaping wounds should be repaired.

If there is doubt about the integrity of the eye, refer.

Conjunctival foreign bodies

Foreign bodies blown into the eye, or loose lashes, commonly lodge in the lower fornix and are easily removed. If the foreign body is under the upper lid, not only does it scratch the cornea with each blink, but it cannot be removed without everting the lid. The steps for doing this are as follows (Figure 5.1):

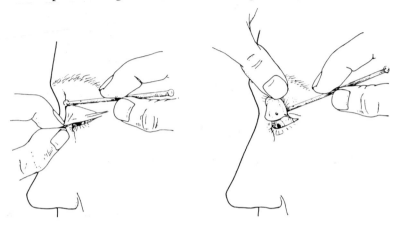

Fig. 5.1   Eversion of upper lid, to remove subtarsal foreign body

1. The patient looks downwards with both eyes open.
2. The operator grasps the eyelashes between finger and thumb of one hand while, with the other, he presses the tip of a pencil, a cotton bud or an unfolded paper clip on the skin of the lid just above the tarsal plate.
3. The foreign body is removed.
4. The cornea is stained with fluorescein (p. 3). If an abrasion is found, antibiotic ointment should be used.

The upper and lower fornices of the conjunctiva are surprisingly capacious, and quite large foreign bodies may be concealed there.

Subconjunctival haemorrhage (Figure 5.2)

A localized haemorrhage may follow injury to the eye and often is part of an orbital haematoma. The blood is absorbed in a week or two, but, if severe, the condition should raise suspicion of more serious injury such as fracture of the orbital walls or penetrating injury of the globe.

Spontaneous subconjunctival haemorrhage, often recurrent, is common in in the elderly, and is sometimes associated with

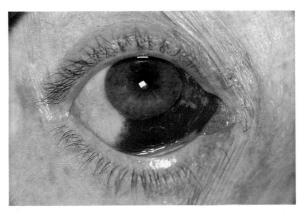

Fig. 5.2 Subconjunctival haemorrhage (spontaneous)

hypertension, clotting disorders, or conditions associated with increased venous pressure.

Chemical injuries of the conjunctiva

Energetic first aid may be crucial after exposure to corrosive chemicals. Workers in chemical industries or laboratories may receive splashes of liquid acids or alkalis in the eyes. Although reflex tear production dilutes the irritant, immediate irrigation of the eyes with abundant water may be a sight-saving measure. The injured person's head should be held under a tap, while companions help to hold the eyes open while water runs over them. Subsequent management depends on the severity of the burning and the nature of the chemical concerned. Alkalis are, in general, more dangerous than acids. Liquid ammonia and caustic soda cause permanent corneal and conjunctival damage and possibly blindness. Any severe case should be referred after immediate first aid.

Lime requires special mention. Lime particles may be splashed in the face, especially of a building worker, when powder flies up during the mixing of cement. There is immediate blepharospasm and lacrimation, making examination difficult. Treatment is as follows:

1. Anaesthetize with 1% amethocaine hydrochloride or 0.4% oxybuprocaine hydrochloride (Minims® Benoxinate (Oxybuprocaine) Hydrochloride).

2. Remove all solid particles of lime from the conjunctiva, using forceps or cotton wool swabs.

3. Irrigate the eye thoroughly with water.

4. Stain with fluorescein.

5. If the cornea is clear and there is no conjunctival necrosis, instil antibiotic ointment.

6. If necrosis is present or the cornea is cloudy, refer.

Conjunctivitis (Figure 5.3)

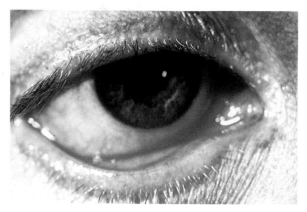

Fig. 5.3   Acute conjunctivitis

Inflammation of the conjunctiva is the commonest ophthalmic problem for the GP. The causes are summarized in Table 5.1. Symptoms are discomfort, discharge, and difficulty in opening the eye on waking. Signs are redness and discharge adherent to the lashes. Hypertrophy of lymphoid follicles may be seen, particularly in the lower fornix where they appear as shiny round swellings. The upper lid should be everted in a search for enlarged papillae on its conjunctival surface. Pre-auricular lymph node enlargement may be present. Visual acuity is not affected unless there is also corneal involvement, but the cornea should be stained with fluorescein and examined with magnification in a good light (see p. 3) to ensure that the epithelium is intact.

Some cases of chronic conjunctivitis defy definitive diagnosis and therapy. Such patients may be referred for assessment by an ophthalmologist.

Table 5.1   Causes and clinical features of conjunctivitis

Cause	Clinical features
Bacterial infection	Mucopurulent discharge, crusting on lashes
Viral infection	Non-purulent ± lower fornix follicles ± corneal lesions No response to antibiotics

Allergy
  Atopic conjunctivitis
  Vernal conjunctivitis
	Marked in pollen season
	History of allergy; itching the main symptom
	Papillae on upper tarsal conjunctiva
	± corneal lesions

Chemical and drug reactions	History of exposure ± lower fornix follicles
Mechanical causes	Eyelid abnormalities Trichiasis Exposure
Dry eye	Rose bengal staining Reduced tear secretion ± associated systemic disorder

Bacterial conjunctivitis

Purulent discharge and difficulty opening the eyes on waking are the cardinal features, with relatively mild, gritty discomfort.

It is helpful to perform a bacterial culture before starting treatment. The bacteria commonly causing conjunctivitis are:

Niesseria gonorrhoeae – onset in <24 hours

Haemophilus influenzae – onset in <3 days

Streptococcus pneumoniae – onset in <3 days

Moraxella lacunata – onset in 3 days or more

Staphylococcus aureus – onset in 3 days or more

Chlamydia trachomatis – characterized by chronicity.

Antibiotic drops – usually chloramphenicol or ofloxacin – should be given for at least 5 days; antibiotic ointment may be given at night, in addition. A sustained-release formulation of fusidic acid, Fucithalmic® viscous eye drops, has been shown in clinical trials to be of equal efficacy to chloramphenicol. The drops are dispensed from a tube, like ointment, which enables a twice-daily dosage to be prescribed.

Chlamydial conjunctivitis (Figure 5.4)

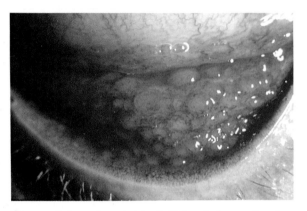

Fig. 5.4   Chamydial conjunctivitis: follicles in lower fornix

Bacteria of the genus *Chlamydia* live only within cells, forming intracellular inclusion bodies. *Chlamydia trachomatis* affects primarily the human eye and genital tract, but any mucous membrane may become involved. Following an acute initial infection, a chronic, often subclinical, phase follows. It should be assumed that a patient with chlamydial conjunctivitis also has a genital tract infection. Systemic treatment is required. Refer, where possible, to a sexually-transmitted diseases clinic after initiating at least topical treatment.

Three distinct clinical syndromes are produced by infection of the conjunctiva by *C. trachomatis*:

1. *Neonatal inclusion conjunctivitis* (see p. 46).
2. *Endemic trachoma* – a chronic infection seen amongst under-privileged people living in warm dry climates with poor standards of hygiene. It is the world's major blinding condition in younger people. Sporadic cases seen in developed countries are usually inactive.

3. *C. trachomatis conjunctivitis* (adult inclusion conjunctivitis) is caused by strains of this organism which infect the genital tract and are transmitted to the eye following sexual contact. The only adults to be affected are sexually-active. *Chlamydia* is the commonest cause of non-specific urethritis in men and of pelvic inflammatory disease in women. The conjunctivitis is florid, predominantly in the lower fornix, with follicle formation and punctate staining of the cornea. It is often unilateral.

The diagnosis is usually made after the condition has failed to respond to first-line treatment for bacterial conjunctivitis. Confirmation may be obtained by microscopy of conjunctival cells, treated with Giemsa's stain or iodine to identify inclusion bodies. Most laboratories now use fluorescent labelled monoclonal antibodies and/or enzyme-linked immuno-absorbent assay (ELISA) instead of culture. A swab is smeared onto a clean microscope slide and fixed with acetone or similar fixative. These methods have the advantage that viable tissue is not required, and have replaced chlamydial culture in most centres.

The treatment is controversial, and advice about 'best practice' changes frequently – one of the reasons for recommending specialist referral. Current management (1997) is as follows:

Systemic. The tetracycline group of drugs are the treatment of choice:

doxycycline 100 mg b.d. for 1 week
or
tetracycline 500 mg q.i.d. for 1 week
or
azithromycin 1 g stat. dose

erythromycin 500 mg q.i.d. for 1 week is the recommended treatment for pregnant or lactating women

Topical. 1% chlortetracycline (Aureomycin® ophthalmic ointment) three times daily (for 6 weeks for a cure) or erythromycin ointment (same regime). Topical treatment will resolve the eye signs, but should not be given without systemic treatment. Cases of doubt should be referred. Questions should be asked about sexual contacts, who should be treated by their GP or a genito-urinary medicine specialist.

Conjunctivitis in the newborn (ophthalmia neonatorum)

This is a notifiable disease and includes any purulent discharge from the eyes within 21 days of birth. Infection occurs during birth and appears within 2 or 3 days as gross oedema of the lids, between which pus escapes when an attempt is made to open the eye. The conjunctiva is congested and swollen (chemosis).

A culture should be taken from any newborn infant with conjunctivitis, and the eyes should be examined to determine the state of the cornea. The organisms commonly found on culture are:

Haemophilus spp.
Neisseria gonorrhoeae
Staphylococcus aureus
Streptococcus pneumoniae
Chlamydia trachomatis

Treatment with ophthalmic chloramphenicol six times per 24 hours usually clears the infection, except in the case of *C. trachomatis*, the treatment for which is Erythroped® syrup – 50 mg/kg body weight divided into four doses per 24 hours, for 3 weeks.

If there is any question of corneal damage, or the infection persists, viral cultures should also be taken and an attempt made to identify *Chlamydia*. Discharge must be cleared with cotton wool. Initial treatment is best carried out as a hospital in-patient.

Viral conjunctivitis

Adenovirus. Typically occuring in epidemics, eye infection by adenovirus is a potentially serious, bilateral disease. There is non-purulent, watery discharge. The conjunctivitis is associated with fine, punctate corneal ulcers and subepithelial opacities and, frequently, pre-auricular lymph node enlargement. The diagnosis can be confirmed by culture using a viral transport medium. The disease usually lasts 2–3 weeks, but symptoms may persist for months or years, with episodes of recurrent keratitis (Figure 5.5).

Strict hygienic precautions must be observed to minimize the risk of transfer of infection, especially in schools and within the family. Treatment is of little value, though symptomatic relief may be obtained from warm compresses, rest and antibiotic drops or agents containing vasoconstrictors, such as Otrivine-Antistin®

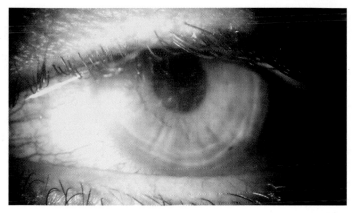

Fig. 5.5   Adenoviral keratoconjunctivitis: note punctate corneal opacities

drops. Patients in whom corneal complications are suspected should be referred for specialist care.

Herpes simplex. Primary herpes simplex infection may cause a short-lived conjunctivitis. Herpes simplex keratitis is discussed on page 60.

Herpes zoster. The affected eye may show marked conjunctival involvement. Management is discussed on page 61.

Other viral infections. Transient non-purulent conjunctivitis is a feature of many systemic viral infections. No specific treatment is required; the watering and redness settle with the resolution of the illness. It is important to check the eyelid skin for previously unrecognized lesions of molluscum contagiosum (see p. 25), which may be the cause of recurrent conjunctivitis which defies treatment with antibiotics.

Allergic conjunctivitis

Allergic conjunctivitis occurs in several distinct forms:

1. *Acute allergic conjunctivitis.* This bilateral condition is an urticarial reaction to allergen reaching the conjunctiva directly. It may appear with dramatic suddenness and subside equally quickly. Treatment, apart from identifying and, if possible, avoiding the cause, is with topical and systemic antihistamines. Steroid drops, instilled every hour or two until the swelling subsides, usually

prove satisfactory. An alternative is the new, highly potent topical histamine H_1 antagonist, levocabastine (Livostin®), applied twice per 24 hours.

2. *Seasonal allergic conjunctivitis.* This is usually a mild, bilateral inflammation with marked itching and no discharge; follicles may be present, particularly in the lower conjunctival fornices. The condition is most evident during the hay fever season. Typically, the cornea is not involved, but the distinction must be made from drug-induced allergic conjunctivitis, where contact lens soaking and cleaning solutions are the cause (p. 126).

Treatment should, where possible, be topical, and the condition can usually be satisfactorily managed in general practice. This is a controversial subject, and the placebo response can be significant. Levocabastine (Livostin®) drops applied twice per 24 hours may give rapid and sustained relief. Mast cell stabilizing drops such as sodium cromoglycate (Opticrom®) drops (four times per 24 hours), or nedocromil sodium(Raptil®) drops (twice per 24 hours) are often effective. Severe cases may require steroid drops; fluorometholone (FML®) is the least likely to cause a rise in intraocular pressure. As with any other use of topical steroids, it is essential that the prescribing doctor checks the cornea for dendritic ulceration by staining with fluorescein before starting treatment. If steroid treatment is continued for more than 4 weeks, the checking of intraocular pressure by accurate tonometry is mandatory. Oral antihistamines such as terfenadine (Triludan®), 60 mg twice per 24 hours during active phases, may also be helpful. A search for causative antigens by skin testing may help the patient.

3. *Vernal conjunctivitis* ('spring catarrh') (Figure 5.6). Typically seen in atopic individuals in childhood and early adult life, the most serious of these IgE-mediated conditions is readily diagnosed by the finding cobblestone-like papillae on the upper tarsal conjunctiva of both eyes on everting the upper lids. Papillae produce elevations of the conjunctival surface, each consisting of a telangiectatic vessel surrounded by dilated capillaries and inflammatory infiltrate. Each papilla can be a millimetre or more in diameter. Numerous eosinophils are found on microscopic examination of the conjunctival scrapings. Corneal complications are common.

Once diagnosed, the condition should be managed under specialist care, but the GP may have to handle periodic exacerbations. Topical steroids such as prednisolone drops 0.5% or sodium cromoglycate (Opticrom®) are of about equal effectiveness. The

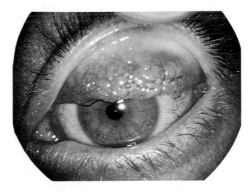

Fig. 5.6 Vernal conjunctivitis: giant papillae on upper tarsal conjunctiva

condition usually resolves in early adult life, but permanent corneal scarring may remain.

Chronic non-specific conjunctivitis

Conjunctivitis which persists despite treatment is common, though seldom disabling. Abnormalities of the eyelids (ectropion and entropion) and trichiasis should be excluded, and tear secretion measured by Schirmer's test (p. 36). Referral to an ophthalmologist seldom results in a curative prescription, but useful reassurance may be obtained. (See Table 2.2, p. 15)

Degenerative conditions of the conjunctiva

Pinguecula (Figure 5.7)

This is a common condition in adults of all ages. Near the corneoscleral junction medially and laterally, areas of subconjunctival degeneration occur, seen as creamy triangular plaques which may be elevated. Occasionally pingueculae become inflamed. Steroid drops remove the redness, but the usual precautions of staining the cornea to exclude ulceration, and avoidance of prolonged use of the drops, must be observed.

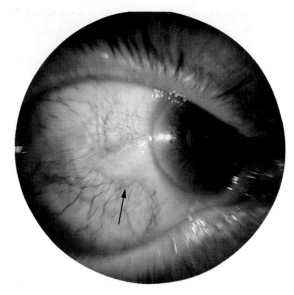

Fig. 5.7   Pinguecula: note that lesion does not invade cornea

Pterygium (Figure 5.8)

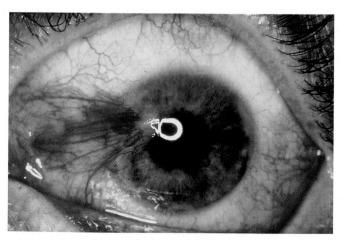

Fig. 5.8   Pterygium: note that lesion invades cornea

This is a wing-like area of subconjunctival degeneration, occuring at the limbus and extending over the cornea. An opaque zone preceding the tip of the advancing pterygium indicates activity. If it is considered unsightly or threatens to cover the pupil, the patient should be referred for excision of the pterygium. A few days of considerable discomfort usually follow excision, and recurrence is possible. The patient should be warned of this.

Tumours of the conjunctiva

These are rare and include the following:

Benign

Papillomata and *cysts* may be simply excised if causing discomfort or cosmetic blemish.

Naevus

Often close to the limbus, a conjunctival mole may be of any colour from coffee to jet black. It is slightly raised and has a nodular surface. Some become larger and darker at puberty. Unless excision is demanded for cosmetic reasons, no treatment is indicated. Any increase in size or vascularity of the lesion – like melanomata elsewhere – should be regarded with suspicion. Malignant change occurs rarely and is an indication for wide excision. Photography is a simple and accurate method of monitoring any change in these naevi.

Malignant

Carcinoma of the conjunctiva is very rare. Malignant melanomata are considered above.

Episclera and sclera

Episcleritis (Figure 5.9)

Inflammation of the episcleral tissue deep to the conjunctiva is usually unilateral, with slight discomfort and no discharge. The eye may be diffusely red or the inflammation localized; there may be an inflamed nodule, usually in the interpalpebral zone. The adjacent conjunctiva is not inflamed.

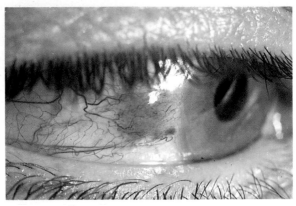

Fig. 5.9 Nodular episcleritis

Although episcleritis may be associated with systemic disorders, it usually occurs for no known reason in healthy individuals and resolves spontaneously in a few weeks.

Treatment with steroid drops such as prednisolone 0.5% four times per 24 hours is helpful. It is important to ensure that the cornea does not stain with fluorescein before starting treatment with steroids.

Scleritis (Figure 5.10)

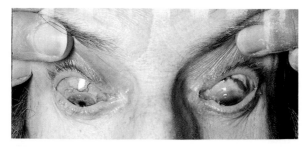

Fig. 5.10 Scleritis: right eye active, with scleral thinning nasally; left eye has gross scleral thinning (scleromalacia)

Inflammation of the sclera is painful and often affects both eyes. The deeper vessels are engorged. Prolonged scleritis leads to scleral thinning, so that the blue of the underlying ciliary body is seen. There may be associated sclerosis of the adjacent cornea, leading to opacification and marginal corneal thinning. Scleritis is usually seen in association with systemic disease, commonly rheumatoid arthritis complicated by vasculitis. The overall incidence of scleritis in patients with rheumatoid arthritis is low, however, and treatment is a matter for a specialist.

6
The cornea

Anatomy

Despite its thinness (about 1 mm), the cornea is remarkably tough. The exposed surface is covered with epithelium continuous with that of the conjunctiva. Beneath the epithelium are numerous free nerve endings, explaining the sensitivity of the cornea and the pain resulting from injury or inflammation.

The corneal stroma is bounded superficially by Bowman's membrane and, on its deep surface, by Descemet's membrane. The innermost layer is the endothelium, important in keeping the cornea optically clear by the transfer of fluid from the stroma into the adjacent anterior chamber against the hydrostatic gradient of the intraocular pressure. The endothelium is of importance to the surgeon carrying out intraocular operations as its cells do not regenerate; they enlarge to cover a greater area and their number diminishes with age, in disease, or after trauma. If the endothelium fails, corneal oedema develops and vision is lost.

Peripherally, the cornea blends with the sclera at the limbus, a specialized region where most of the drainage of aqueous humour takes place. The inner aspect of this area contains the trabecular meshwork, communicating, via the canal of Schlemm, with the episcleral veins on the surface of the globe. This is the main outflow pathway for the aqueous humour.

Congenital and hereditary disease

Keratoconus (conical cornea) (Figure 6.1)

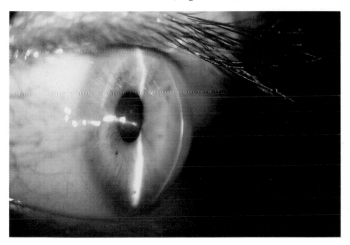

Fig. 6.1   Keratoconus: note also small pterygium

In this condition the cornea, having been normal in childhood, loses its normal curvature. It becomes increasingly steeply curved in early adult life, with resultant irregular refraction of the entering light. Visual acuity falls, and cannot be improved by spectacles. Keratoconus can most easily be demonstrated by observing the lower lid curvature when the patient looks down (Munson's sign).

No medical treatment can arrest the development of keratoconus, but satisfactory vision can often be obtained with rigid contact lenses (see p. 125). If corneal oedema or scarring develops, vision may be restored by corneal grafting.

Corneal dystrophies

This is an obscure group of conditions occurring more commonly in adult life and with a familial tendency. Corneal opacities develop bilaterally and interfere increasingly with vision. There are no inflammatory signs, except in rare superficial dystrophies in which there is recurrent corneal erosion. The pathological process cannot be reversed by medical treatment, but corneal grafting usually produces improvement.

Fuchs' dystrophy is of particular importance in the elderly. It is a degenerative condition with affects the endothelium, with a tendency to corneal oedema when the endothelial cells are no longer able to maintain corneal clarity. When associated with cataract, Fuchs' dystrophy presents a difficult problem for the surgeon, who is faced with the need to carry out both cataract extraction and full-thickness corneal grafting. Fuchs' dystrophy may recur after grafting.

Congenital limbal dermoid

This congenital, non-progressive tumour occurs at the corneal margin and covers a variable extent of the cornea. It is pearly-white, elevated, and may have hairs on its surface. Excision is often required on cosmetic grounds, though a permanent scar remains.

Trauma

Corneal abrasion

This is an injury involving the epithelium. There is pain, lacrimation, photophobia and blepharospasm. The diagnosis is confirmed by staining the cornea with fluorescein (Figure 6.2). Examination is easier if the eye is anaesthetized with a drop of local anaesthetic. If there is a possibility of a foreign body, a thorough search of the conjunctival sac, with eversion of the upper lid (see p. 40) is necessary.

Treatment is with antibiotic ointment and a firmly applied pad until the epithelial defect has healed – normally within 24–48 hours. Infection and failure to heal will lead to corneal ulceration.

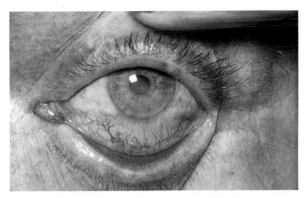

Fig. 6.2   Corneal abrasion, stained green with fluorescein

Recurrent corneal erosion

Apparently trivial corneal injuries may lead to the intermittent recurrence of symptoms. A mother whose eye is injured by her baby's finger is typical. Following healing of the initial abrasion, the patient wakes from sleep with pain because an area of unstable epithelium has been shed on first opening the eye. Symptoms subside during the day, as adjacent epithelial cells slide over to cover the defect. This sequence is repeated at intervals.

Plentiful application of a non-steroid ointment at night for a month or two is usually effective: Lacri-Lube® ointment, obtainable without prescription, is suitable. Alternative treatments involve removal of the affected area of epithelium with alcohol, after anesthetizing the cornea, or the use of a soft, 'bandage' contact lens for an extended period. Difficult cases should be referred for confirmation of the diagnosis by slit-lamp examination, and for specialist advice about management.

Welder's flash ('arc eye')

Welder's flash and snow blindness are similar conditions and are due to exposure to ultraviolet light. After an interval of 6 or 8 hours, intense bilateral lacrimation, blepharospasm and photophobia develop. Examination may not be possible until the eyes have been anaesthetized with 1% amethocaine hydrochloride. Once the blepharospasm has been relieved, multiple punctate corneal erosions are seen to stain with fluorescein. The lesions heal within a few hours.

Local anaesthetic drops and reassurance are the only treatment required.

Foreign bodies

Usually there is a clear history of the entry of a foreign body, though other irritants, such as a loose lash or a subtarsal foreign body, cause similar symptoms.

A good light and magnification help removal. A drop of local anaesthetic such as 1% amethocaine hydrochloride is instilled and the foreign body removed. If it is loosely adherent to the cornea, it may be removed with a cotton bud or the corner of a tissue. A sterile 17-gauge needle is a convenient instrument to pick a foreign body off the cornea. Antibiotic ointment is used four times per 24 hours for 4 days, and the patient reports back if the eye is uncomfortable or the vision blurred. Mydriatics are usually unnecessary: atropine, with its prolonged action, is never required. Following the removal of a metallic foreign body, a rust ring may remain; this is more readily removed after 2 or 3 days' use of antibiotic ointment.

Patients should be advised about protective measures.

Perforations of the cornea

All perforations, and cases in which there is suspicion, should be referred, and the patient instructed to take nothing by mouth in order to be ready for general anaesthesia. Normal visual acuity may be consistent with the presence of an intraocular foreign body. A history of hammering metal on metal, with no evident super-ficial foreign body, suggests an intraocular metallic fragment, and the finding of a subconjunctival haemorrhage heightens suspicion. Radiography of the eye usually demonstrates a metallic foreign body, however small.

Laceration of the cornea causes a reduction in depth of the anterior chamber as compared with the other eye, or distortion of the pupil. Injury to deeper structures may be seen as lens opacities or haemorrhage in the eye (see p. 80).

Early detection is of great importance in successful management. Damage to the eye by a retained intraocular foreign body, by infection, or by resulting retinal detachment, may be irreversible. 'Missed' intraocular foreign bodies are an unfortunate but regular cause of justified medico-legal claims. If there is any suspicion of penetration, refer to hospital.

Corneal inflammation (keratitis)

A corneal ulcer is usually painful. There may have been previous episodes of corneal ulceration or other eye disease, or a history of a foreign body or trauma. The cause of corneal ulceration may be bacterial, fungal, a foreign body, viral, exposure or toxic reaction. If contact lenses are worn, they should be suspected as having a role in the development of any keratitis.

Visual acuity is reduced if the central cornea is involved. Fluorescein staining and inspection in good light will show the size, situation and shape of any ulcer.

Bacterial keratitis

Infection usually enters the cornea after injury. The eye is painful, photophobic and watery. There is a sensation of something in the eye due to movement of the lids over the epithelial defect. The eye is red, most markedly in the quadrant where the ulcer lies. Visual acuity is usually reduced. A greyish area of oedema and opacity may be seen before stain is used. Fluorescein demarcates the edges of the ulcer. A search should be made for a foreign body on the cornea, or under the upper lid.

Before starting treatment it is important to identify the causative organism. This involves performing cultures and taking a direct scraping from the ulcer bed for urgent microscopic examination. These cases should be referred.

Treatment should be under specialist supervision. Intensive topical antibiotic applications are needed, usually combined with a mydriatic such as atropine 1%. Hospital admission may be desirable. Padding the eye is usually unnecessary. Failure to heal within 48 hours or so, or the development of a level of pus – a hypopyon – within the anterior chamber, are indications for urgent referral.

Marginal keratitis (Figure 6.3)

This represents a local hypersensitivity reaction to conjunctival infection by certain organisms, usually *Staphylococcus aureus*. Conjunctivitis may be slight, but there is photophobia, pain and vascular congestion at the limbus, where round or elongated ulcers, or subepithelial corneal infiltrates, are found. These features do not progress centrally.

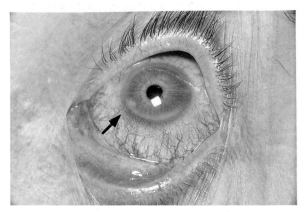

Fig. 6.3   Marginal keratitis with associated bacterial conjunctivitis: note white corneal infiltrate

In addition to treating the conjunctivitis with antibiotic drops or ointment, a topical steroid may be used. This is one of the few ophthalmic situations where the use of combined antibiotic/steroid is justified over a short time, provided that no dendritic ulcer is present (see below).

Viral keratitis

Herpes simplex keratitis (dendritic ulcer)

This infection is primarily confined to the corneal epithelium, and the resultant dendritic ulcer is a common and serious condition. It presents as an irritable eye (often without much discomfort) and is diagnosed after fluorescein staining (Figure 6.4) as a branching ulcer. The virus lies dormant in the trigeminal nerve between attacks.

Treatment is with a topical antiviral agent. Of several available, the most effective and least toxic is acyclovir (Zovirax®) ointment, used five times per 24 hours until the ulcer has healed. This should be under specialist supervision, but initial treatment may be started by the GP as soon as the diagnosis is made.

Recurrence is common, and is treated in the same way. Steroid preparations should never be used in general practice if herpes simplex infection is suspected.

Complications. Amoeboid ulceration is a more advanced form of the disease, in which the ulcer spreads to assume a confluent pattern. Treatment is with antiviral agents.

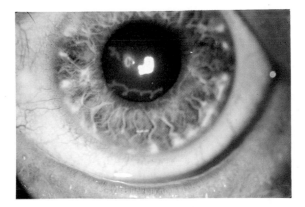

Fig. 6.4   Dendritic ulcer, stained with fluorescein

Disciform keratitis and kerato-uveitis. Herpes simplex infection of the deeper layers of the cornea leads to central corneal thickening and opacification, described as 'disciform keratitis'. There is usually associated uveitis. Treatment is difficult and needs to be carefully monitored in a specialist unit; frequently, diluted steroid drops are used at the same time as an antiviral agent. Activity may last for months. Permanent scarring of the cornea is common and may necessitate corneal grafting. Fortunately, herpes simplex keratitis is usually unilateral.

Herpes zoster (Figure 6.5)

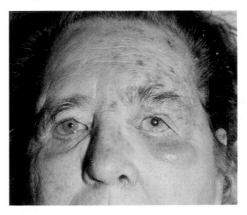

Fig. 6.5   Herpes zoster ophthalmicus: note vesicles on left side of nose and dependent oedema of lower lid

Corneal ulceration may occur during the acute stage of ophthalmic herpes zoster; conjunctival inflammation, uveitis and secondary glaucoma are also seen, as is a dendritic-like ulcer. Vesicles appearing on the tip of the nose indicate involvement of the external nasal branch of the ophthalmic division of the fifth cranial nerve, and suggest eye involvement. Later, corneal sensation may be impaired and lid deformities occur, resulting in a chronic keratitis which is difficult to manage.

Treatment is controversial and may be difficult. The patient may be ill and unwilling to attend an eye clinic. On first appearance of the skin eruption, oral antiviral agents have proven efficacy in minimizing post-herpetic neuralgia. Acyclovir (Zovirax®) 800 mg tablets are given 4-hourly, omitting the night-time dose, for 7 days – alternatively, valaciclovir (Valtrex®) 500 mg, two tablets given three times per 24 hours, or famciclovir (Famvir®) 250 mg, three tablets daily as a single dose for 7 days. The once-daily dose helps with compliance. Adequate hydration must be maintained, particularly in the elderly. These treatments are expensive.

There is no general agreement as to what to apply to the affected skin; it is probably best to put on nothing at all – the infection is in the nerves, not the skin. A simple ointment will keep the skin supple and relieve local discomfort, but topical antiviral skin creams do not play any significant role.

Topical treatment of the eye should consist of acyclovir five times per 24 hours for 5 days, or until the eye is white. If it is suspected that the eye is involved, the patient should be referred, but it is important to start treatment as soon as possible. It may be difficult to open the lids, but a relative or nurse should be able to get some ointment into the conjunctival sac.

Swelling of the subcutaneous tissues around the other eye is not a cause for concern. This is usually due to tissue fluid which tracks across the midline in a patient who lies in bed with the affected side uppermost.

Analgesics will generally be required: co-proxamol, dihydrocodeine or buprenorphine are all suitable. Systemic prednisolone, 80 mg daily, reducing over 1 week, is recommended only for patients with neurological complications (see below).

Complications, apart from eye and lid inflammation and their direct sequelae, include extraocular muscle paralysis (most commonly involving the third cranial nerve), optic neuritis and hemiparesis. Post-herpetic neuralgia may be a long-term problem, but seems to be less severe in patients treated with oral antiviral agents. Herpes zoster infection in patients with impaired immunity, either from disease or from the use of immunosuppressive drugs, is likely to be more prolonged and severe; hospital admission is essential. Hospital admission should also be considered for any patient in whom the eye is involved.

Adenoviral keratitis

This epidemic condition is discussed under conjunctival infections (p. 46).

Fungal keratitis

Injuries, particularly by vegetable matter, occasionally cause corneal ulcers which are resistant to conventional antibiotic treatment. Necrotic material seen in the ulcer bed may prove to contain fungi.

In common with other situations in which corneal ulcers fail to respond to antibiotics, referral is essential.

Other forms of keratitis

Acanthamoeba keratitis

Acanthamoeba is a protozoon commonly found in soil and water. It may infect the cornea – contact lens wearers are most at risk, accounting for 80% of cases. Poor hygiene practices, notably the preparation at home of non-sterile saline solutions and the rinsing of contact lenses with tap water, are important causes of infection.

The infection produces severe, painful ulceration of the cornea, which is refractory to antibiotics. The organism can be demonstrated by microscopy and culture. Diagnosis and management are a matter for the specialist.

Keratoconjunctivitis sicca

See Chapter 4, p. 36.

Neuroparalytic keratitis

Loss of corneal sensation deprives the cornea of one of its protective mechanisms and may be followed by ulceration. In addition to herpes zoster affecting the ophthalmic division of the fifth cranial nerve (see p. 61), any lesion of this nerve which produces corneal anaesthesia may lead to keratitis. Protection of the cornea, by the copious use of ointment at night and spectacles with protective side-pieces, may be sufficient. Patients at risk of corneal ulceration should be referred: tarsorrhaphy (temporary or permanent partial closure of the lids), or 'bandage' soft contact lenses may be required. A temporary tarsorraphy, lasting up to 2 weeks, can be achieved with histoacryl glue (superglue). This should be only be undertaken by a specialist.

Rosacea keratitis (Figure 6.6)

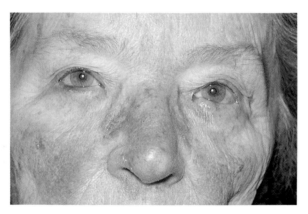

Fig. 6.6   Rosacea: note posterior blepharitis, right lower lid

Rosacea leads to reddening of the skin of the face, telangiectasia and episodes of inflammation. The cause is unknown. Corneal involvement begins with marginal vascular infiltration; ulceration and opacification may follow.

Treatment with low-dosage oral tetracycline (250 mg b.d. between meals), or doxycycline 100 mg daily, for at least 2 months usually controls exacerbations.

Possible ophthalmic complications are posterior blepharitis, chalazia, conjunctivitis and keratitis.

Bell's palsy

Idiopathic facial palsy may lead to exposure keratitis. While waiting for recovery of movement, the patient should be supplied with plenty of antibiotic ointment to put in the affected eye at night. Taping the lids together at night is often helpful. If recovery is delayed for more than 2 months, particularly if the eye is uncomfortable or persistently red, referral for a lateral tarsorraphy is appropriate.

Dysthyroid exophthalmos

Proptosis due to this or any other cause may place the cornea at risk from exposure. Dysthyroid eye disease is considered on p. 171. Plenty of ointment at night is the first measure, reinforced, if necessary, by taping the lids (see above).

Other causes of exposure keratitis

Any debilitating disease may lead to the patient sleeping with imperfectly-closed eyes (lagophthalmos), with consequent drying of the cornea – seen as a lack of normal lustre in the epithelium. Ointment should be instilled regularly. In severe cases, padding of the eyes, with a paraffin gauze square under the pad, may be necessary until normal lid closure returns.

Degenerative conditions of the cornea

Band-shaped opacity

In some degenerate eyes and in those which have sustained previous injury or inflammation, a horizontal opacity develops in the interpalpebral portion of the cornea, with deposition of calcium in its superficial layers. Patients with this condition should be referred. Treatment with chelating agents applied under local anaesthesia may be considered.

Pterygium (Figure 5.8)

This is a degenerative condition arising in the conjunctiva and extending horizontally as a wing-like opacity of the cornea. It may need surgery (see Ch. 5).

Material for corneal grafting

The extension of organ transplantation to include kidney, liver, heart and lungs, and the problem of transmissible virus diseases (particularly hepatitis and AIDS, and also the slow virus diseases affecting the central nervous system), have made corneal grafting dependent on organ donor centres. Fortunately it is now possible to store donor cornea for extended periods, making corneal grafting a procedure which can be undertaken on a planned basis.

In the United Kingdom the service is centralized at The United Kingdom Transplant Service, Southmead Road, Bristol BS10 5ND, telephone 01179 757575, to which enquiries should be directed.

7
The middle coat of the eye

Anatomy

The vascular, pigmented middle coat of the eye – the uveal tract – is in three parts – iris, ciliary body and choroid. The iris diaphragm lies against the lens, separating the anterior and posterior chambers of the eye. The ciliary body produces aqueous humour and permits variation of focus of the eye (accommodation) through its attachment to the lens by the zonular fibres. The ciliary muscle is innervated by the parasympathetic component of the third cranial nerve.

The sphincter pupillae (parasympathetic, third cranial nerve) and dilator pupillae (cervical sympathetic) control the size of the pupil. The highly vascular choroid and the central retinal artery together nourish the retina.

Congenital abnormalities

Aniridia

Congenital absence of the iris is a rare, genetically-determined abnormality. Affected individuals are likely to have poor vision and to develop glaucoma. Aniridia is part of a spectrum of uncommon disorders of the anterior segment of the eye, collectively known as mesodermal dysgenesis.

Albinism

Pigment is absent from the eye (ocular albinism) or from the whole body. Vision is poor and nystagmus occurs. Albinoid children should be referred for specialist assessment.

Colobomata (Figure 7.1)

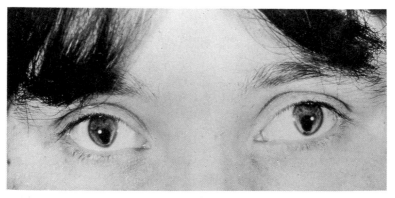

Fig. 7.1 Iris colobomata

Incomplete closure of the fetal choroidal fissure of the developing eye leaves a defect – a coloboma – in the uveal tract, in its lower nasal quadrant. Colobomata extending posteriorly in the choroid may be associated with poor vision.

Trauma

Non-perforating eye injuries (due to squash balls, shuttlecocks, etc., which are small enough to enter the orbit) may damage the uveal tissues.

Hyphaema (Figure 10.1) (see Ch. 10)

Bleeding into the anterior chamber causes blurred vision. When the blood has settled, a level is seen in the anterior chamber. Patients with hyphaema are usually referred to hospital because of the possibility of secondary haemorrhage: though uncommon, this can be disastrous. Contusion severe enough to produce hyphaema frequently causes damage to the anterior chamber angle, and may lead to glaucoma years later (p. 157).

If a patient with traumatic hyphaema is not admitted to hospital, rest should be advised until the blood has been absorbed.

Traumatic mydriasis

Paralysis of the iris sphincter following contusion may lead to a persistently dilated pupil; there may also be impairment of accommodation. Recovery after a few weeks is common.

Iridodialysis

This is a tear of the iris root.

Choroidal tear

Force from a contusion injury transmitted to the posterior segment of the eye may result in a crescentic tear of the choroid, usually temporal to the disc. Severe visual impairment may result; there is no treatment.

Uveal inflammation

Suppurative inflammation of the uveal tract is usually obvious and requires urgent referral. Non-suppurative uveitis, an important cause of blindness, is more difficult to diagnose and remains poorly understood. Although occasionally secondary to other ocular disorders, including keratitis and cataract, most cases of uveitis are endogenous.

Acute anterior uveitis (iritis) (Figures 7.2a and 7.2b)

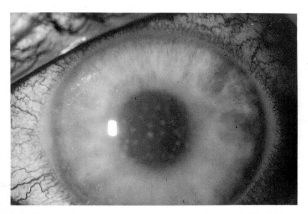

Fig. 7.2a   Acute iritis, showing keratic precipitates and ciliary and iris vessel congestion

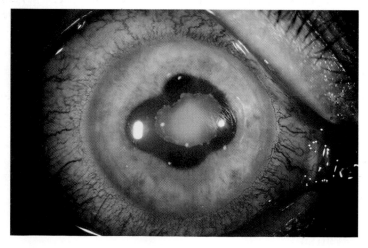

Fig. 7.2b   Acute iritis, showing ciliary congestion, posterior synechiae causing pupil distortion, and exudate on lens surface

This is the form of uveitis most important in general practice. Presenting as a red and photophobic eye, it is usually unilateral and is sometimes associated with patients who have differing iris colouration. There is engorgement of the blood vessels around the limbus. The pupil is small and may be irregular, due to the inflamed iris becoming adherent to the anterior lens surface, and producing adhesions known as posterior synechiae. Frequently, visual acuity is impaired. Clumps of leucocytes adhering to the posterior surface of the cornea (keratic precipitates) may be seen under magnification. Keratic precipitates and posterior synechiae are diagnostic of uveitis. Exact diagnosis may, however, be difficult. All suspected cases should be referred urgently.

The cause, in most cases, cannot be found, although about half have the HLA B27 antigen. Systemic disorders such as seronegative arthritis, sarcoidosis, ankylosing spondylitis and Reiter's disease may be found in patients with iritis.

Treatment is with topical corticosteroids used every 2 hours, and cyclopentolate hydrochloride 1% or atropine 1% to dilate the pupil. Steroids, either systemically or by injection round the eye, are required if drops fail to control the inflammation. Recurrences are common. A patient known to have had uveitis and who presents again to his GP may be treated initially with steroid drops and a mydriatic, provided examination of the cornea (with fluorescein) has shown no dendritic ulcer to be present.

Posterior uveitis (choroiditis, chorioretinitis) (Figure 7.3)

This condition is painless and the eye is usually white. Blurred vision or the finding of fundus lesions at routine ophthalmoscopy are the usual modes of presentation.

Most cases are of unknown cause, and treatment is correspondingly haphazard and unrewarding. Systemic granulomatous conditions such as sarcoidosis, tuberculosis and syphilis are occasionally found in patients with posterior uveitis.

Two specific conditions with which posterior uveitis may be associated deserve mention:

1. Toxoplasmosis

This may be either congenital or an acquired infection. The former is of significance in the eye, but the acquired disease, which may occur at any age, usually causes no ocular symptoms.

In congenital toxoplasmosis, the causative organism has a predilection for central nervous tissue and, in the extreme form, causes severe brain damage. Convulsions may be the first symptom, and intracranial calcification may be evident on X-ray examination of the skull. Ocular toxoplasmosis produces scarring in the retina and choroid – a white lesion surrounded by accumulated black pigment in the inactive stage (Figure 7.3). Such a focus at the posterior pole prevents the development of macular vision.

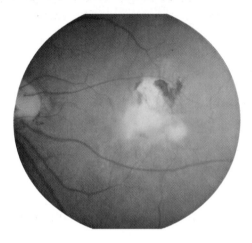

Fig. 7.3   Toxoplasmic chorioretinitis: superior portion of lesion shows old scarring; inferior portion shows active inflammation, where margins are indistinct

Toxoplasmosis lesions in the eye may undergo apparently spontaneous reactivation, producing signs of posterior uveitis, often with associated inflammation in the anterior segment. Cloudiness of the vitreous causes blurred vision; visual loss is profound if the reactivated focus lies near the macula or optic disc.

Diagnosis is usually made on clinical grounds, but antibody tests such as the toxoplasmosis dye titre may help.

Treatment is unnecessary unless vision is impaired, but any patient known to have ocular toxoplasmosis who notices blurred vision should be referred. Steroids by mouth or by intraorbital injection are usually combined with an antimicrobial agent such as clindamycin 300 mg four times per 24 hours for some weeks. Pseudomembranous colitis is a rare but serious side effect of this drug.

2. Toxocariasis

Infection of the eye by the nematode worm *Toxocara canis* is an uncommon but serious form of posterior uveitis, usually occurring in young children who play on ground contaminated by the faeces of puppies which have not been 'wormed'. The parasite reaches the posterior pole of the eye, producing a chorio-retinal lesion which irreversibly destroys central vision. Fortunately, it is generally unilateral. Presentation usually results from routine visual acuity testing or the detection of a squint. Treatment has little to offer.

Acquired immune deficiency syndrome (AIDS)

See p. 109 and Figure 9.15.

Tumours of the uveal tract

Iris

Tumours of the iris are rare, but any patient concerned that a tumour may be developing should be referred for a specialist opinion.

Ciliary body

Malignant melanoma occasionally develops in the ciliary body, causing distortion of the pupil or detachment of the retina. These tumours, if not too large, may be treated by local resection, resulting in the preservation of useful vision.

Choroid

Benign naevus (Figure 7.4)

These flat, pigmented areas usually occur in the posterior half of the fundus. They are seldom significantly elevated and there is no associated retinal detachment. Distinction between larger naevi and malignant tumours may be difficult. Cases of doubt should be referred for observation and investigation, which may include fluorescein angiography, serial fundus photography, and B-scan ultrasonography (see p. 185).

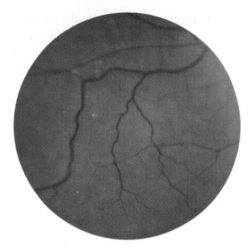

Fig. 7.4   Benign choroidal naevus

Malignant melanoma (Figure 7.5)

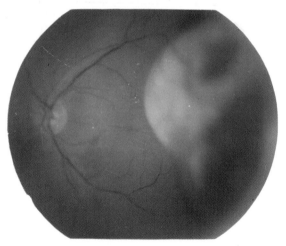

Fig. 7.5   Malignant choriodal melanoma

These tumours arise anywhere in the uveal tract – iris, ciliary body or choroid. Iris melanomata must be distinguished from the commonly occurring benign naevi. They seldom grow aggressively, but if malignancy is suspected the tumour should be excised with a segment of iris.

Malignant melanoma of the ciliary body and choroid is a life-threatening condition. The lesion is elevated and tends to cause an associated retinal detachment, with peripheral field loss and, later, impairment of central vision. Distant metastases are common and a search must be made for evidence of metastatic spread when planning treatment.

Treatment is controversial: patients treated by enucleation have been shown to be at greater risk of dying from metastases in the years immediately following surgery than those left untreated. However, the prospect of extrascleral extension cannot be viewed with equanimity. Local resection of the tumour with preservation of the eye is sometimes feasible, as are various forms of radiation therapy. Patients over 70 years old are sometimes left untreated if the tumour is small.

Metastatic tumours

These tumours present similarly to malignant melanoma, but their growth is more rapid. Palliative radiation may be justified. Tumours arising from breast carcinoma usually respond to tamoxifen.

8
Cataract

Any opacity in the lens is a cataract. Many are either non-progressive or increase only slowly; only a small proportion eventually need surgical treatment. However, cataract is the commonest single reason for referral by GPs to ophthalmologists and its treatment forms the largest part of the surgical workload of most Eye Departments.

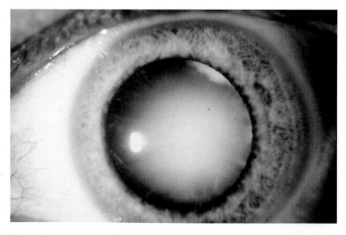

Fig. 8.1 Cataract, predominantly nuclear

Lens opacities can occur within any part of the lens. A central, or nuclear, cataract (Figure 8.1) often presents as an amber-coloured opacity when viewed with the slit-lamp, whereas the less common posterior cortical opacity appears more like a lace curtain at the posterior surface. Peripheral cataracts may have no optical significance and can usually be ignored.

Most commonly patients are referred to their GP by the optometrist, who has found a fall in visual acuity and the presence of lens opacities. The GP will be involved in deciding when to refer a patient with cataract, when the medical and social situations have been considered. The GP may also participate in the postoperative management, particularly with regard to the recognition of posterior capsule opacification. An understanding of the issues involved is therefore essential.

Classification of cataract

1. Congenital
2. Cataract associated with other disorders
   a. metabolic
   b. syndromes of multiple congenital deformity
   c. skin disease
   d. drugs
   e. physical causes: trauma, heat, ionizing radiation, electric shock, previous intraocular surgery
   f. secondary to other eye disease
3. Senile.

Congenital cataract

The lens develops by the infolding of a vesicle from the surface ectoderm. Within this vesicle, layers of lens fibres develop, the oldest being forced towards the centre and the youngest being found on the surface. Interference with this process results in opacity. For example, rubella, during the first trimester of pregnancy, conveys a definite risk of the child being born with congenital defects in the eye (and also in the ear or heart). Cataract due to rubella is a sporadic disorder; many congenital cataracts are familial.

Incomplete congenital cataracts are known as lamellar (zonular) cataracts. While the majority of congenital lens opacities do not increase after birth, some types, particularly of a punctate variety, become more dense in later life and may then require surgery.

The presence of an opaque lens in the eye of an infant is an absolute indication for referral within the first few days of life if there is to be any prospect of useful treatment. Total removal of the cataractous lens, together with the anterior part of the vitreous – lensectomy – is usually the operation of choice. Optical correction can subsequently be provided by 'soft' contact lenses suitable for long-term wear. Close supervision is essential or amblyopia (p. 143) will negate the benefits of surgery. Retinal detachment, often many years after surgery for congenital cataract, is an important potential complication and must be taken into account when deciding whether to advise operation.

Cataract associated with other disorders

Metabolic

1. *Diabetes mellitus*. Diabetics develop cataract at an earlier age than non-diabetics, and cataract patients attending eye clinics are routinely examined for glycosuria. In one study, 3% of patients were found to have diabetes, previously undiagnosed. The management of cataract in diabetics does not differ from that in non-diabetics, but postoperative complications are rather more common and removal of a dense cataract may reveal diabetic retinal changes.

2. *Galactosaemia*. Cataracts in newborn infants with galactosaemia are reversible by early treatment.

3. *Hypocalcaemia*. Cataract, characteristically of the subcapsular type, may follow hypocalcaemia from any cause.

4. *Dystrophia myotonica* – a condition of unknown cause, in which a metabolic defect is presumed. The condition generally becomes apparent at 20–30 years of age and progresses slowly. Patients have a typically expressionless facial appearance with a slow, unrelaxing smile and bilateral ptosis. Other features include frontal baldness and genital atrophy. There is widespread neurological abnormality, characterized by inability to relax muscle groups – most strikingly found in the handgrip. The patient becomes slow and apathetic.

There is no known treatment for the underlying disorder. Visual impairment by cataract is usual by 40 years of age, but the results of cataract surgery are good.

Syndromes of multiple congenital deformity

In Down's syndrome, characteristic cataracts appear at about the age of puberty.

Skin disorders

Cataract is associated with certain disorders of the skin, e.g. atopic dermatitis.

Drugs

Steroids given over long periods, topically or systemically, may cause cataract – typically of the posterior subcapsular type, which interferes markedly with vision.

Physical causes

1. *Trauma.* Injury to the lens capsule leads to opacification of lens fibres due to exposure to aqueous. A small hole in the capsule may lead to limited opacity, but more severe injury leads to rapid opacification of the entire lens, which may swell, causing secondary glaucoma. Contusion, without rupture, can cause a characteristic rosette-like cataract, progressing rapidly to total opacity.

Treatment depends on the age of the patient, any associated injury and the state of the fellow eye. Surgery is usually indicated.

2. *Radiation.* Infrared, microwave and ionizing radiation, and severe electric shock may cause cataract.

Secondary to other eye disease

Long-standing eye disorders such as chronic uveitis and persistent retinal detachment commonly lead to cataract.

Senile cataract

This is the most important category of cataract: 50% of people over 80 years of age have significant cataract. Senile cataract is usually bilateral, though progression may be faster in one eye than the other. The exact biochemical cause of opacification of the lens is unknown.

Symptoms

The patient complains of failing vision. Apparently sudden deterioration may be due to a long-standing defect only recently noticed. The rate of progress is unpredictable. Patients with cataracts of the nuclear sclerosis type, which cause an increase of refractive index of the nucleus of the lens, present with increasing myopia. Such patients, supplied with a presbyopic spectacle correction for reading, may enjoy a period in which they can read unaided.

Diagnosis

Visual acuity is reduced. A 'pin-hole' test (p. 8) will eliminate refractive errors as the cause of the visual loss. The diagnosis is made by examination of the eye with an ophthalmoscope through a dilated pupil. A cataract is most easily seen from a distance of about 50 cm with a +3 lens in the ophthalmoscope: the red reflex in the pupil is broken by opacities within the lens.

Surgical treatment

Indications

With the rare exception of galactosaemia in infants, non-surgical treatment of cataracts is not of proven benefit. Cataract surgery may be considered for any patient whose vision is significantly reduced in one or both eyes. There is no absolute level of acuity at which surgery should be advised or withheld. Occasionally cataracts can produce rapid changes in refraction, with the need for frequent changes of spectacle lenses, known as index myopia – this may be an indication for surgery despite relatively good vision. Maturity of a cataract is a strong indication for its removal; a light directed obliquely at the pupil casts a shadow in the pupil unless the cataract is fully mature, when the entire pupil appears opaque. Complications, including lens-induced uveitis and glaucoma, are likely in the presence of an untreated mature cataract.

Approach

The enormous change in cataract surgery since the 1970s has been the development of intraocular lenses to compensate for the absence of the natural crystalline lens (aphakia). Intraocular lenses are now used in practically all cases except where there is a specific contraindication, e.g. in chronic uveitis. Even high myopes benefit from the provision of a lens which accurately corrects the eye to a satisfactory postoperative refractive state. The power of the lens implant required to give the desired postoperative refraction can be determined by biometry (p. 185).

Patients for whom lens implants are considered unsuitable must use alternative optical correction, by rigid or soft contact lenses (Ch. 11) or 'aphakic' spectacles.

Techniques

A detailed discussion is inappropriate, but there are two regularly-used methods of cataract removal.

1. *Phakoemulsification* (Figures 8.2a and 8.2b). An incision less than 4mm long is made in the peripheral corneal or sclera. After removal of a disc of anterior lens capsule (capsulorrhexis), the lens is fragmented with a phakoemulsifier and the lens matter aspirated through the coaxial handpiece. A rigid or folding lens implant is introduced through the same incision. Usually no sutures are needed. Recovery of vision is frequently almost instantaneous.

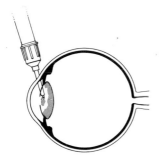

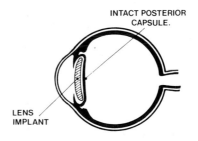

INTACT POSTERIOR CAPSULE.

LENS IMPLANT

Fig. 8.2a Cataract extraction: lens matter removed from within lens capsular envelope by phakoemulsification

Fig. 8.2b Lens implant: note intact posterior lens capsule behind posterior chamber lens implant

2. *Extracapsular extraction.* This is a similar technique to phakoemulsification, but a larger incision is needed to express the lens nucleus. The anterior lens capsule is incised, the nucleus expressed, the cortex aspirated, and an implant inserted, usually into the capsular envelope. The capsule remaining in front of the implant is then removed and the eye sutured with fine mono-filament nylon. These sutures may be selectively removed in the follow-up period if they are causing distortion of the eye and astigmatism; otherwise, they dissolve 2 or 3 years later. Glasses are prescribed after 6–8 weeks, when the wound healing has stabilized.

Anaesthesia can be either topical, usually with peri- or retro-bulbar injection of a long-acting agent and with or without basal sedation, or general, if preferred by the patient or surgeon. The operation is usually undertaken as a 'day-case' procedure. No patient need be considered too old or frail for cataract removal.

Follow-up

The advice given to the patient after cataract surgery is a matter for the individual surgeon, but the GP is likely, from time to time, to become involved.

The recovery period after surgery, whether undertaken as an in-patient or day-case, is about 6 weeks, after which eye drops are no longer needed and definitive glasses are prescribed. Any patient with a painful or discharging eye, particularly with worsening vision, may have an intraocular infection and should be referred back to hospital forthwith. Such cases are, happily, rare. It is not unusual for the eye to be inflamed and mildly irritable post-operatively. Most surgeons prescribe steroid/antibiotic eye drops for the first few weeks following surgery, and the GP will be asked to renew this prescription as necessary.

Traditionally, postoperative cataract patients were advised not to stoop, have their hair washed, and so on; these restrictions are unnecessary with phakoemulsification or modern suturing techniques. Patients are now advised to avoid vigorous activity, such as digging the garden and moving heavy furniture, but most elderly cataract patients need simply to be a little careful during the first few weeks. They may drive, providing they are comfortable and have adequate vision.

Outcome

Both surgical techniques give excellent results. In a national cataract surgery survey conducted in the UK in 1990, the proportion of patients without coexisting ocular pathology which had achieved 6/12 or better acuity 3 months after surgery was 75–96%, depending on age group.

Posterior capsule opacification (Figure 8.3)

It is essential for the GP to understand that, following cataract surgery in which the posterior lens capsule is preserved, the capsule may subsequently become opaque. This change may be regarded more as part of the healing process than as a complication of surgery, but its effect is to produce gradual deterioration of vision in an eye which, after the operation, had good sight. Posterior capsule opacification is more common in younger patients, and less so after 70 years of age.

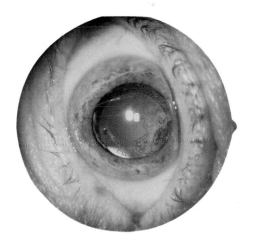

Fig. 8.3 Posterior capsule opacification after laser capsulotomy: note diamond-shaped capsular opening behind lens implant

The GP must be vigilant and refer patients whose vision has deteriorated months or even years after successful cataract surgery. This applies particularly to the older and less articulate. They may otherwise become increasingly and unnecessarily blind in the belief that, having undergone surgery, nothing further can be done.

Treatment

Posterior capsule opacification is readily treated by YAG laser capsulotomy. This is an out-patient procedure. It is best postponed until at least 3 months after cataract surgery. Capsulotomy in the first few months after surgery leads to a higher incidence of serious complications, such as retinal detachment and cystoid macular oedema, than if it is carried out later.

Once the posterior lens capsule has been adequately opened by laser, it will not become opaque again. The cause of subsequent visual loss is likely to be in the retina (Ch. 9).

Suture disintegration

Nylon sutures used to close the incision after extracapsular extraction may become loose or disintegrate at any time up to several years postoperatively. Fine nylon sutures are often invisible to the naked eye, but easily seen with a slit-lamp. The patient complains of discomfort or a watering eye, which may be red. Referral to the hospital or surgeon quickly solves the problem.

9
The retina and vitreous

Anatomy
- Retina
- Vitreous

Arteriosclerotic and hypertensive retinopathy

Hypertension
- Haemorrhages
- 'Hard' exudates
- Retinal infarcts
- Optic disc oedema

Vascular occlusion and haemorrhage
- Central retinal artery occlusion
- Retinal branch arterial occlusion
- Amaurosis fugax
- Central retinal vein occlusion
- Retinal branch vein occlusion
- Vitreous haemorrhage

Macular disorders
- Genetically-determined macular disorders presenting in childhood
- Macular disorders in early adult life
- Myopic macular degeneration
- Age-related macular degeneration
- Other macular disorders

Drug toxicity in the retina

Diabetic retinopathy
- Management
- Classification

Retinopathy of prematurity (retrolental fibroplasia)

Retinal detachment
- Diagnosis
- Management

Retinal detachment without a retinal break

Retinoschisis

Eclipse burn of the macula

Inherited disorders of the retina
- Retinitis pigmentosa

Tumours of the retina

Inflammatory disorders of the retina
- Acquired immune deficiency syndrome (AIDS)
- Other inflammatory disorders

Anatomy

Retina

The retina develops as an outgrowth of the forebrain, which is invaginated to form two layers. The outer layer becomes the retinal pigment epithelium and the inner layer the sensory retina, with the rods and cones adjacent to the pigment epithelium and the nerve fibre layer innermost.

At the posterior pole is an oval area some 5 mm in diameter – the macula. This contains a yellowish pigment. It is only at the macula that detailed visual discrimination, such as reading fine print, is possible. The central area of the macula, the fovea, contains cones, but no rods. The fovea lies about 3 mm temporal to the optic disc. The healthy fovea gives a bright light reflex when seen with an ophthalmoscope. At its centre, the fovea has a depression 0.4 mm in diameter – the foveola. Here the cones have no overlying layer except the internal limiting membrane.

The blood supply of the retina is from the central retinal artery, except at the fovea where the tissues are nourished from the innermost layer of the choroid – the choriocapillaris. The central retinal artery divides into four main branches, each accompanied by a tributary of the central retinal vein. The diameter of each vein exceeds that of the corresponding artery in a 3:2 ratio. Where they cross there is, in the normal fundus, no interference with the alignment of either vessel.

Vitreous

The vitreous is a transparent gel with a collagenous fibrillary structure, occupying the posterior segment of the globe. In the healthy eye of a young person the vitreous is in contact with the entire retina, being attached at its anterior extremity (the ora serrata) and at the optic disc. Passing across the vitreous from the disc to the posterior lens surface is the embryonic hyaloid vessel system.

With ageing, particularly in myopic eyes, the vitreous undergoes liquefactive change – syneresis. In the elderly, the periphery of the vitreous commonly becomes detached from the retina and optic disc, and the hyaloid remnants are visible to both patient and observer as large 'floaters'.

Arteriosclerotic and hypertensive retinopathy

Arteriosclerosis may develop in the retinal vessel walls (Figure 9.1). The changes are most obvious at the arteriovenous crossings: the arterial walls lose their transparency and obscure the view of the underlying vein on either side of the column of blood. Further changes lead to pallor of the arterial light reflex, more marked crossing changes, greater tortuosity of the larger vessels and a change of alignment at the crossing from the normal oblique angle towards a right angle. The vein distal to the crossing may be dilated.

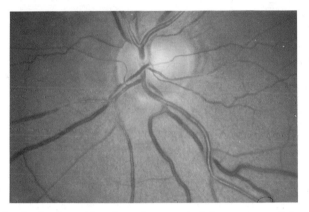

Fig. 9.1   Retinal arteriosclerosis: note heightened arteriolar reflex and arterio-venous crossing changes

Advanced arteriosclerosis shows as marked pallor of the arterial light reflex and irregularity of the lumen, with yellowish staining of the vessel walls, like the stem of a clay pipe. The blood column disappears completely in places. In extreme cases the vessels may appear to be completely occluded, though their patency can be shown by angiography.

Hypertension (Figure 9.2)

Younger hypertensive patients show narrowing of the arterioles. Prolonged hypertension leads to structural changes in the vessel walls, the hypertrophied smooth muscle being replaced by fibrous tissue. Older patients in whom there is significant arteriosclerosis show arteriovenous crossing changes and irregularity of arterial calibre. More severe hypertension may result in further retinal changes: haemorrhages, 'hard' exudates, retinal infartcs ('cotton wool' spots, formerly termed 'soft' exudates) and optic disc oedema.

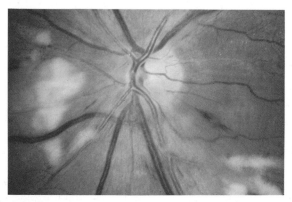

Fig. 9.2   Hypertensive retinopathy: note haemorrhages and 'cotton wool' spots

Haemorrhages

Retinal haemorrhages in hypertension are most frequently seen in the superficial, nerve fibre layer of the retina. They may be linear or flame-shaped, and are most numerous near the optic disc. Haemorrhages confined to one sector of the fundus signify local-ized retinal vascular occlusion (see p. 92). Haemorrhages seldom interfere with vision unless there is macular involvement.

'Hard' exudates

'Hard' exudates are yellowish-white deposits in the deeper layers of the retina. They represent accumulated fat deposits and the residue of oedema. Their size varies from small dots to areas with a diameter greater than that of the disc. They are commonly found in the region between the disc and the macula and in a star forma-tion around the macula.

Retinal infarcts

'Cotton wool' spots are retinal infarcts in the nerve fibre layer, and are indicative of ischaemia. They are accumulations of degenerate axoplasm. 'Cotton wool' spots occur in the most severe forms of hypertensive retinopathy and indicate a grave prognosis. They are also seen in other systemic disorders, for example, diabetes (see p. 98), collagen disorders, blood dyscrasias and the acquired immune deficiency syndrome, AIDS (p. 109).

Optic disc oedema

Since the classification of hypertensive retinopathy by Keith, Wagener and Barker (1939), oedema of the optic disc has been regarded as the surest indication of severe hypertension. Optic disc oedema, 'cotton wool' spots and flame-shaped haemorrhages indicate accelerated ('malignant') hypertension. The coexistence of other features of hypertensive retinopathy and the relatively slight elevation of the optic disc help to differentiate this condition from papilloedema, which is due to raised intracranial pressure.

Vascular occlusion and haemorrhage

Central retinal artery occlusion

Failure of the retinal circulation leads to sudden and profound visual loss. This is an emergency, and the patient should be referred immediately to an Accident and Emergency Department. If the occlusion persists, the ischaemic retina sustains irreversible damage, with swelling of the inner retinal layers due to the accumulation of degenerate axoplasm. Usually occurring in the elderly, central retinal artery occlusion may be due to an embolus from the carotid or to thrombosis of an already arteriosclerotic vessel.

The presenting symptom is sudden, painless loss of vision in one eye. Examination shows the absence of direct pupillary light reaction and pale, attenuated retinal vessels. With progressive retinal damage, generalized retinal oedema is seen, except at the macula. Here the retina is thinnest and the area appears as a reddish spot owing to the visibility of the underlying choroidal circulation.

Unless the occlusion is caused by an embolus which subsequently passes into a more peripheral vessel, relieving the central obstruction, visual loss is permanent and optic atrophy becomes apparent after a few weeks. The retinal oedema subsides. There may be an audible carotid bruit.

The investigation of central retinal artery occlusion should include the following investigations: blood pressure; urinalysis; ECG; chest and skull radiography; and duplex carotid ultrasonography or i.v. digital subtraction angiography (selective carotid angiography). Carotid blood flow may alternatively be investigated by carotid artery imaging (see ch. 17). Blood should be analyzed for the following: full blood count; ESR/viscosity; glucose; urea; syphilis serology and lipids.

Management of central retinal artery occlusion in the first few minutes consists of attempting to lower the intraocular pressure to encourage the onward passage of any embolus. Firm massage of the globe through the closed lids is probably the most effective treatment available to the GP. The patient should be referred for ophthalmological assessment and review of the carotid arteries and cardiovascular system.

Retinal branch arterial occlusion

Also presenting as sudden, painless loss of vision, the portion of the visual field lost depends upon the extent of retinal arterial closure (Figure 9.3).

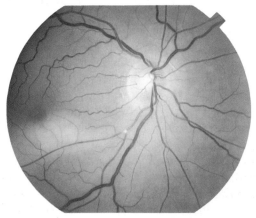

Fig. 9.3   Retinal arteriolar occlusion: note embolus at bifurcation of inferior temporal branch and oedema of affected sector of inferior retina

Amaurosis fugax

Transient occlusion of the central retinal artery or one of its branches gives rise to 'fleeting blindness'. The patient usually complains of a 'curtain' obscuring vision for a few minutes. This is a form of transient ischaemic attack and is often the precursor of a major cerebrovascular accident. An embolus may be visible in one of the retinal arterioles. Giant cell arteritis (p. 160) is a less common cause: the diagnosis depends on finding a raised ESR, and can be confirmed by temporal artery biopsy.

A carotid bruit should be sought by auscultation over the carotid bifurcation, at the level of the upper border of the larynx. Significant carotid stenosis may be present in the absence of a bruit and non-invasive techniques are available to study flow and turbulence: these include duplex carotid ultrasonography and intravenous digital subtraction angiography. Selective intra-arterial cerebral angiography is seldom indicated; it entails a risk of disabling stroke of about 1%.

Aspirin 300 mg daily is often recommended to reduce the likelihood of further transient ischaemic episodes. Attention must be paid to the control of all risk factors for stroke and myocardial infarction, including hypertension and smoking habits.

Central retinal vein occlusion

Occlusion of the vein has a less sudden presentation than that of the artery, owing to the variable element of ischaemia that accompanies venous obstruction. Visual loss is usually profound, developing over a period of hours or days.

The fundus appearance (Figure 9.4a) is typically dramatic, with extensive haemorrhages throughout, often as if red paint had been thrown at the retina; there may be numerous 'cotton wool' spots. Secondary, neovascular glaucoma may occur about 3 months later (p. 157), due to the growth of new blood vessels which progressively occlude the drainage angle. New retinal vessels may develop and subsequently give rise to vitreous haemorrhage.

Central retinal vein occlusion is predominantly a disease of the elderly. More than 60% of patients with this condition have high blood pressure, and generalized cardiovascular disease and diabetes are also commonly found. Raised intraocular pressure, with or without established open-angle glaucoma, is also an important aetiological factor of central retinal vein occlusion.

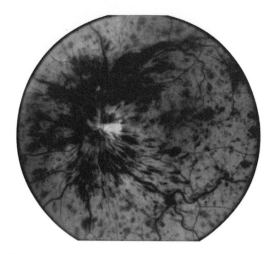

Fig. 9.4a   Central retinal vein occlusion

Haematological factors such as dysproteinaemias and blood dyscrasias may also have a role, and oral contraceptives may be a contributory cause.

Every case of central retinal vein occlusion should be referred for ophthalmological assessment as well as medical screening. The ophthalmologist may investigate the degree of ischaemia in the retinal circulation by fluorescein angiography (p. 184), to help to decide whether laser treatment is likely to prevent secondary thrombotic glaucoma. The most important aspects of the patient's management are the correction of hypertension and other treatable circulatory and biochemical disorders.

Retinal branch vein occlusion (Figure 9.4b)

Occlusion of part of the retinal venous circulation occurs more commonly than central vein occlusion, and usually affects one of the vessels on the temporal side. Occlusion is distal to a crossing point, and haemorrhages and 'cotton wool' spots are confined to the affected area of the fundus. If the macula is involved, central vision will be affected; otherwise the condition may pass unnoticed by the patient and be found at a routine fundus examination.

The aetiology is the same as that of central retinal vein occlusion, and the patient should be similarly referred for investigation.

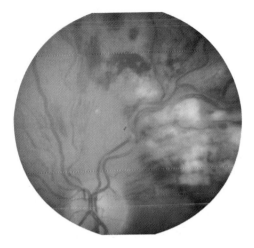

Fig. 9.4b   Retinal branch vein occlusion: 'cotton wool' spots indicate retinal ischaemia in affected sector

Vitreous haemorrhage

The symptoms of vitreous haemorrhage vary from the appearance of a few spots before the eye to sudden, complete, and painless visual loss. The diagnosis is made by finding blood in the vitreous on examination with a 'plus' lens in the ophthalmoscope – or by being able to see nothing at all with the instrument, if the haemorrhage is severe and the vitreous totally opaque.

Vitreous and other intraocular haemorrhages may occur spontaneously in perfectly healthy people, especially on severe exertion or the performance of a Valsalva manoeuvre. Trauma is also an important cause. Apparently spontaneous vitreous haemorrhage needs urgent referral, in case there are other abnormalities within the eye.

Diabetes, hypertension and blood dyscrasias must be excluded, and the patient investigated to identify treatable vascular disease. A full fundus examination should be carried out by an ophthalmologist at the earliest opportunity. If retinal details cannot be seen satisfactorily, the patient should be kept under periodic review until, with clearance of the haemorrhage, a view of the fundus is obtained. Ultrasound investigation is of value in vitreous haemorrhage as a means of excluding underlying retinal detachment.

A number of retinal disorders may present with haemorrhage into the vitreous, including a retinal tear or detachment, retinal vein occlusion or localized vascular abnormality. New vessel formation associated with vein occlusion, diabetes, sickle cell disease or retinal vasculitis may be found. Diagnosis is a matter for the ophthalmologist.

Persistent vitreous haemorrhage may be treated surgically, by vitrectomy.

Macular disorders

Macular disorders may profoundly impair central vision but leave peripheral, navigating vision unaffected. The patient's symptoms will alert the GP to the likely cause, but he/she may not have available sufficiently detailed examination techniques to make a confident diagnosis, and most cases will therefore need to be referred. Pupillary dilatation with a short-acting mydriatic such as tropicamide 0.5% is essential for a satisfactory view of the macula.

An acute macular disturbance will usually impart kinks to straight lines, and make objects seem smaller (micropsia) or larger (macropsia) than they appear with the other eye, owing to displacement of the foveal cones. The pupillary light reaction is unaffected – in contrast to disorders of the optic nerve, in which there may also be profound loss of visual acuity with preservation of the peripheral visual field (see p. 162).

Patients with severe bilateral macular degeneration of any type usually maintain a fairly high level of independence; navigational vision is likely to remain satisfactory. Appropriate advice and support are helpful and reassuring. For information on blind and partially-sighted registration, see page 191.

A complete list of macular disorders is inappropriate, but they may be classified according to likely age of onset.

Genetically-determined macular disorders presenting in childhood

The commonest in this group of rare disorders is Stargardt's macular dystrophy. Children with initially normal vision show progressive impairment of acuity to 'counting fingers' in their second decade, and characteristic yellowish lesions appear at the posterior pole. Inheritance is recessive and both sexes are equally affected. Management consists of the provision of visual aids.

Macular disorders in early adult life

Central serous chorioretinopathy typically affects males, and presents with impairment of vision in the third and fourth decades. Full recovery is usual, though many cases relapse – some repeatedly. The cause is leakage of fluid through a defect in the layer beneath the retinal pigment epithelium, Bruch's membrane. The diagnosis may be confirmed by fluorescein angiography. Laser treatment is sometimes helpful in persistent cases.

Serous detachment of the retina, localized at the macula, may be associated with other ocular disorders, e.g. a pit in the optic disc.

Myopic macular degeneration

High myopes are prone to various retinal disorders, including profound central visual impairment due to degenerative change at the macula, which may result in haemorrhage (Figure 9.5). The choroid and retina become progressively atrophic and extensive areas of white sclera are exposed to view with the ophthalmoscope. It is usually difficult to examine the fundus of a highly myopic eye with a direct ophthalmoscope, but a better view may be obtained if the patient wears his glasses.

Macular degeneration is unlikely to be treatable, but it is important to exclude retinal detachment involving the macula, and referral is therefore essential.

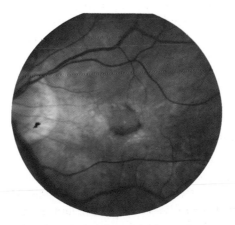

Fig. 9.5 Macular haemorrhage: note also exposed crescent of sclera temporal to disc – a feature of myopia

Age-related macular degeneration (Figures 9.6a and 9.6b)

Age-related macular degeneration (ARMD) is the commonest reason for blind registration in developed countries.

Disciform macular degeneration

This is a common form of age-related macular degeneration, and is usually preceded by the appearance of yellow spots known as colloid bodies. Abnormal new vessels grow beneath the retina from the choroid and these leak, producing subretinal fluid. The consequent visual impairment is made worse by scarring, so that acuity is eventually reduced to 'hand movements'.

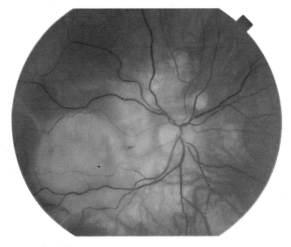

Fig. 9.6a   Age-related macular degeneration, disciform type: right eye of 71-year-old, V.A.: 'hand movements'

If the condition is recognized at an early stage and new vessels away from the fovea are identified by fluorescein angiography, the condition may be treatable by laser, preventing otherwise inevitable deterioration in vision. Successfully treated cases are uncommon, and the likelihood of the second eye becoming involved is about 20% per annum (i.e. it will almost certainly be involved within 5 years). The doctor should therefore warn the patient that symptoms arising in the second eye should be investigated early. Some ophthalmologists give patients already affected in one eye a test card known as an Amsler chart, to check the central vision weekly.

The whole disciform process evolves over a few weeks.

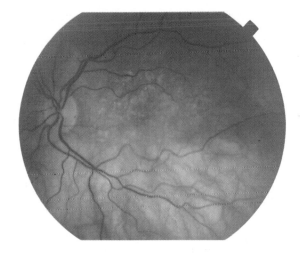

Fig. 9.6b   Age-related macular degeneration, colloid bodies: left eye of patient pictured in Fig. 9.6a, V.A.: 6/9

Macular hole

This age-related condition becomes bilateral in only about 10% of cases. Acuity is reduced to about 6/60. Some cases can usefully be treated by vitrectomy, so referral is appropriate.

Retinal pigment epithelial detachment

This is a more benign form of macular degeneration than the disciform type, but cannot be treated. A change of glasses may help, as the eye becomes relatively more hyperopic. A fibrous scar or an atrophic area at the posterior pole of the eye is the likely outcome.

Other macular disorders

Epiretinal membrane

An epiretinal membrane, giving the retina a characteristically glistening 'cellophane' appearance, may occur after vascular episodes or inflammation, or without apparent cause. There is distortion of central vision and partial loss of acuity, but generally the condition is not progressive. Surgical treatment is sometimes feasible.

Cystoid macular oedema

Cystoid macular oedema may occur in diabetic retinopathy and after retinal vein occlusion (p. 91). Following cataract surgery, it is frequently a transient event of little significance, though it may persist. Treatment is unsatisfactory and the visual outcome uncertain.

Drug toxicity in the retina

Retinal damage may result from the prolonged administration of certain drugs, particularly chloroquine and some phenothiazines. Quinine may cause rapid bilateral visual loss, with dilated, unreactive pupils. Recovery in a few days is usual.

Diabetic retinopathy (Figures 9.7–9.11)

The exact cause of diabetic retinopathy is not known, but experimental and clinical evidence shows that it is in part related to diabetic control. Never seen at the onset in young diabetics, retinopathy has an increasing incidence the longer the duration of diabetes, and on average takes between 7 and 10 years to develop following diagnosis of the diabetes. In the elderly, maturity-onset diabetes may present as retinopathy or its complications before other symptoms of diabetes occur.

The underlying abnormality is in the walls of the small vessels in the retina, leading to local formation of microaneurysms, vessel leakage, exudation and capillary closure. Retinal ischaemia results in new vessel formation. The sight is damaged by oedema; exudation at the macula; haemorrhage arising from damaged and abnormal blood vessels; or by retinal detachment resulting from fibrosis of new vessels and traction on the retina.

Management

Although the prevention of retinopathy may be impossible, good control must always be the aim in managing diabetic patients. Until more satisfactory metabolic management of diabetes prevents retinopathy and the other vascular complications elsewhere in the body, regular, informed review of the fundi and referral for laser treatment as described below are the doctor's essential duty to his diabetic patients.

All diabetic patients, except juvenile-onset diabetics with disease of less than 5 years' duration, should have an annual examination. After testing the visual acuity, the pupils of both eyes should be dilated with a short-acting mydriatic (e.g. tropicamide 0.5%), and a careful fundus examination performed. If significant retinopathy is found, the interval between examinations should be reduced to 6 months.

Any case in which retinopathy is other than 'background' or whether either eye shows 'sight-threatening' features should be referred for further assessment. Visual acuity can in no way be used as a benchmark for the severity of any type of diabetic retinopathy. Early treatment is far more effective than late, and it is of little use waiting for the patient to lose central vision in one eye before referring. Hypertensive and ischaemic changes may complicate diabetic retinopathy. Again, if in doubt, refer.

Laser photocoagulation is now widely available, and its introduction has fundamentally changed the management of diabetic retinopathy and made vigilant observation essential. Diabetics who are pregnant need to be monitored with particular care, as rapid severe deterioration of their retinopathy can occur.

Classification

The object of any classification of diabetic retinopathy is to indicate:
- The present state of the retinopathy
- The need for treatment
- The likely prognosis.

A classification of diabetic retinopathy is summarized in Figure 9.7. The exact terminology is controversial.

1. *'No' retinopathy*. A normal appearance of the fundi in diabetes is a safe indication that no retinal treatment is needed, at least until next year's follow-up. However, fluorescein angiography of apparently normal eyes frequently shows extensive changes not visible on ophthalmoscopy, so there is little room for complacency. Angiography is not necessary routinely.

2. *'Background' retinopathy* (Figure 9.8). The earliest ophthalmoscopic changes in diabetic retinopathy are microaneurysms and haemorrhage. Microaneurysms appear as tiny red dots. The

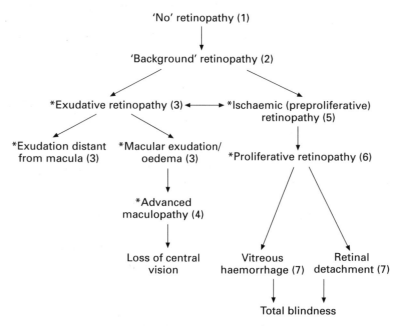

'No' retinopathy (1)

↓

'Background' retinopathy (2)

*Exudative retinopathy (3) ⟷ *Ischaemic (preproliferative) retinopathy (5)

*Exudation distant from macula (3)   *Macular exudation/ oedema (3)   *Proliferative retinopathy (6)

*Advanced maculopathy (4)

Loss of central vision   Vitreous haemorrhage (7)   Retinal detachment (7)

Total blindness

*Indicates sight-threatening retinopathy

Fig. 9.7   Classification of diabetic retinopathy (numbers refer to the text on pp. 99–103)

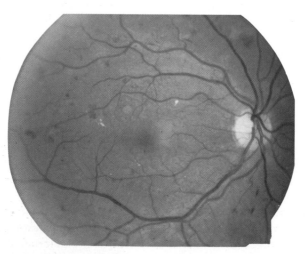

Fig. 9.8   Background diabetic retinopathy

haemorrhages are characteristically of the 'dot' and 'blot' type, which lie in the deeper layers of the retina. 'Hard' exudates are also seen, though if they appear near the macula the classification of the fundus should be exudative maculopathy and the patient referred. 'Background' retinopathy should be followed up every 6 months by the doctor managing the patient's diabetes.

3. *Exudative retinopathy/maculopathy* (Figure 9.9). Significant 'hard' exudates constitute grounds for referral, particularly if they are near the macula. Typically, exudates accumulate in rings around a central area of microvascular leakage. Treatment of this area with laser coagulation usually causes the exudation to regress. Retinal tissue damaged by 'hard' exudates does not recover its function, even though the exudation may disappear – hence the need for treatment before the onset of visual impairment.

Macular oedema may be difficult to detect in the absence of 'hard' exudates. Vision is impaired. Laser applications to the macula, in a grid pattern, may reduce oedema.

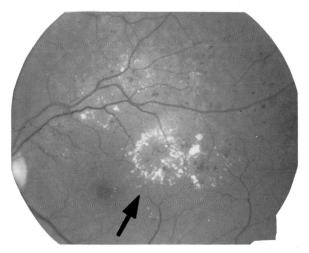

Fig. 9.9   Exudative diabetic retinopathy: arrow indicates ring of exudation surrounding area of microvascular disturbance and capillary leakage

4. *Advanced exudative retinopathy.* Irreversible damage to the macula results in permanent loss of central vision. The patient becomes eligible for blind registration if both eyes are affected, as in advanced senile macular degeneration, but useful 'navigating'

vision is retained. Regular observation is still required, in case the retina develops signs of proliferative retinopathy.

5. *Ischaemic (preproliferative) retinopathy* (Figure 9.10). The signs of impending new vessel formation in the retina – and later the iris and anterior chamber (rubeosis iridis), with its disastrous consequences – are those of ischaemia of the tissues. 'Cotton wool' spots and distension of the veins into sausage-like segments and the formation of loops are the cardinal signs. Any suspicion of these changes or the appearance of new vessel networks, either on the optic disc or elsewhere, demands urgent referral for laser treatment.

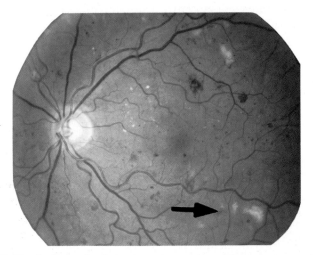

Fig. 9.10   Ischaemic diabetic retinopathy with macular oedema: note distension of infero-temporal vein, 'cotton wool' spots inferiorly, and loss of macular detail

Treatment usually consists of the application of multiple laser burns (3000 or more) to the retinal periphery. The resulting overall reduction in the metabolic requirements of the retina removes the stimulus to new vessel formation, so that already-developed new vessels regress and no more appear. The treatment is an out-patient procedure, often given over several sessions. Follow-up is likely to be carried out in the ophthalmic clinic after laser treatment.

6. *Proliferative retinopathy* (Figure 9.11). New vessels, initially in the plane of the retina and subsequently growing forwards into the vitreous, are seen on the optic disc or elsewhere in the fundus.

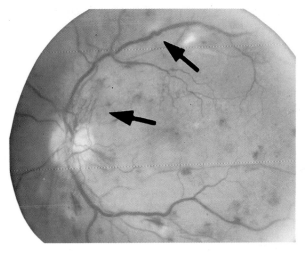

Fig. 9.11   Proliferative diabetic retinopathy: arrows indicate new vessels and a venous loop

The appearance of new vessels indicates urgent need for referral and laser treatment. Failure to treat the retinopathy adequately at this stage leads almost inevitably to loss of vision.

7. *End-stage proliferative retinopathy.* Vitreous and subhyaloid haemorrhage and retinal detachment are disasters requiring referral. The usual practice with vitreous haemorrhage is to examine the eye by ultrasound B-scan (p. 185) to determine whether or not the retina is detached, and to wait for the haemorrhage to clear spontaneously. If it does not, and the ophthalmologist considers that the state of the underlying retina justifies surgery, the blood may be cleared by vitrectomy and the retina treated by photocoagulation from within the eye. Both this, and the surgical treatment of diabetic retinal detachment resulting from traction, by vitrectomy techniques are last-ditch procedures. Blindness resulting from proliferative retinopathy is, unlike the exudative type, usually complete.

Retinopathy of prematurity (retrolental fibroplasia)

Now rare in its fully developed state, retinopathy of prematurity reached epidemic proportions in the 1940s, before its cause was understood. In common with proliferative diabetic retinopathy, abnormal new vessels grow forward from the retina in response to ischaemia.

The administration of oxygen to premature babies with respiratory distress, resulting in high arterial P_{O_2}, causes retinal vasoconstriction; if maintained, this becomes irreversible in 3–4 weeks. On reducing the oxygen concentration in the baby's environment, proliferative changes occur in the retinal circulation.

Infants thought to be at risk are now usually examined by an ophthalmologist before discharge from the neonatal Intensive Care Unit. The peak incidence of abnormalities is at about 7 weeks after delivery. Most cases regress spontaneously, but more severe forms may be treated by cryotherapy or laser. Since the predisposing factors have been better understood, progression to retinal detachment and blindness is exceptionally rare.

Retinal detachment

A common treatable cause of blindness, retinal detachment is of importance to the GP because he/she may be consulted by patients with early symptoms, when prompt referral and early treatment are all-important. The GP must, therefore, recognize the symptoms and signs.

The condition is misnamed. The detachment is that of the sensory retina (rods and cones) from the underlying pigment epithelium, with fluid accumulation between these parts of the retina – inaccurately termed 'subretinal' fluid. Detachment is usually associated with one or more breaks in the sensory retina (Figure 9.12).

Diagnosis

Predisposing factors are myopia, particularly in the middle-aged, previous trauma, cataract surgery and a family history of retinal detachment.

Warning symptoms are flashing lights, associated with increased 'floaters', and spots before the eye. Retinal detachment causes a visual field defect corresponding to the area detached. The patient may complain of a 'curtain' across the vision. Any patient presenting with these symptoms should be sent for urgent examination by an eye surgeon, even if no retinal detachment is seen. Spots before the eye may signify a small vitreous haemorrhage if a

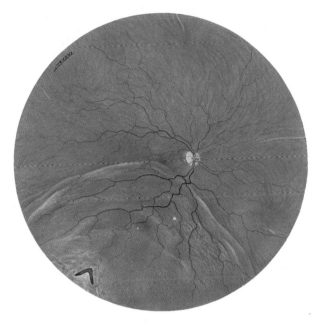

Fig. 9.12   Retinal detachment, with arrow-head retinal break

retinal break passes across a blood vessel. When examined through a dilated pupil, the detached retina appears greyish-blue and may be ballooned forward into the vitreous, the vessels appearing blacker than those on the normal, attached retina.

The diagnostic problem in patients with symptoms suggestive of retinal detachment but no central visual loss is to distinguish 'innocent' degenerative vitreous changes from retinal breaks or early retinal detachment. Responsibility for this should be passed by the GP to the ophthalmologist, who has at his/her disposal more effective techniques for examining the peripheral retina, sometimes a very difficult task.

Management

The retinal breaks are identified and are sealed surgically, either by applying an 'explant' (silicone plomb) to the sclera over the break, or by vitrectomy and internal tamponade; cryotherapy is usually applied to create a permanent seal. Provided the macula is not involved at the start of treatment, excellent restoration of vision is possible in about 90% of cases. Established macular detachment inevitably leads to some impairment of function. Detachment of the superior retina, threatening to involve the macula, demands the most urgent surgical attention and the patient should lie flat until this can be achieved, to prevent inferior extension of the detachment.

The patient should be able to return to work about 6 weeks after retinal detachment surgery, but contact sports and knocks on the head should be avoided indefinitely.

Retinal breaks without detachment may constitute a threat. The ophthalmologist must assess the risk and, where necessary, apply laser or cryotherapy to the breaks or other signs of retinal degeneration. Retinal breaks indicate a significant risk of detachment in the second eye, which should always be examined carefully and, if necessary, treated prophylactically.

Retinal detachment without a retinal break

Intraocular tumours, particularly malignant melanomata, may cause retinal detachment below the tumour. The detachment is likely to be the presenting feature by causing loss of vision, the tumour itself having previously been unnoticed.

Exudative, serous retinal detachment may occur in systemic disorders, e.g. renal failure, and in ocular inflammatory disorders such as scleritis.

Retinoschisis

In contrast to retinal detachment, retinoschisis is a split developing between the layers of the sensory retina. The photoreceptors remain in contact with the underlying pigment epithelium. The condition is not rare. It generally does not progress beyond the equator of the eye, and seldom requires treatment. Cases are found by optometrists at routine refraction examination. It is advisable to seek specialist confirmation of the diagnosis.

Eclipse burn of the macula

Rarely occurring now, ill-advised observation of an eclipse of the sun produces a macular burn sufficient to reduce central vision permanently. Careless handling of a laser may cause a similar disaster.

Inherited disorders of the retina

Retinitis pigmentosa (Figure 9.13)

Retinitis pigmentosa is the commonest of a group of disorders, often with systemic associations, presenting with night blindness and progressive visual field loss.

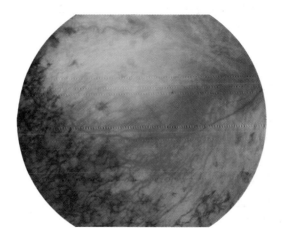

Fig. 9.13   Retinitis pigmentosa: note 'bone corpuscle' equatorial pigmentation and vessel attenuation

Inheritance

Retinitis pigmentosa may be transmitted as an autosomal dominant, recessive or X-linked recessive. About 50% of cases arise with no previous family history; most are probably autosomal recessive.

Presentation

Night blindness is the first symptom, usually appearing in childhood. The more severely affected patients, typically with recessive inheritance, become aware of visual field loss in their second decade. Fundus changes are visible. Progressive field loss makes these patients blind by their fourth of fifth decade, although less severe forms of the disease may not interfere with vision until old age. Cataract may be a complicating factor.

Diagnosis

The fundus appearance is characteristic, with 'bone corpuscle' pigment clumping, particularly in the mid-periphery of the retina, attenuation of the retinal vessels and waxy pallor of the optic disc. Special testing of dark adaptation and of the electrical activity of the retina enable a diagnosis to be made in cases of doubt.

Management

No treatment is effective, but patients may be helped by suitable counselling, retraining and aids for the partially-sighted or blind. Contact with the Retinitis Pigmentosa Society (see p. 193) may be of comfort to many patients, and genetic counselling should be made available to those who request it. Patients with retinitis pigmentosa should generally not drive.

Tumours of the retina

Retinoblastoma is a rare and potentially lethal tumour which may arise by spontaneous mutation or be inherited as an autosomal dominant. The diagnosis is usually made in the first 6 months of life by the appearance of a white mass in the pupil (Figure 9.14) or a squint. Any child with a persistent squint or a white mass in the pupil should be referred, the latter urgently.

Although conservative treatment may be possible, enucleation of the affected eye is usually necessary unless the diagnosis is made when the tumour is small. Regular follow-up during the next 5 years is essential for the early detection and treatment of tumours arising in the fellow eye; about 30% of these tumours are bilateral.

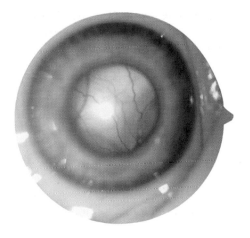

Fig. 9.14   Retinoblastoma

Inflammatory disorders of the retina

Acquired immune deficiency syndrome (AIDS)

AIDS is a multisystem disorder caused by infection with the human immunodeficiency virus (HIV), and involvement of most parts of the body has been recorded. The ocular adnexa may be involved by Kaposi's sarcoma. As the CD4 + T-lymphocyte count declines, the incidence of ophthalmic complications increases.

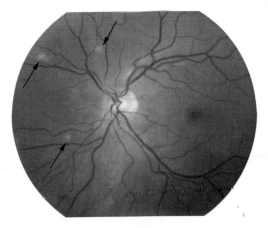

Fig. 9.15   AIDS: arrows indicate 'cotton wool' spots

'Cotton wool' spots in the fundus are the commonest finding (Figure 9.15). Their cause is unknown and they do not interfere with vision. Less common, with a prevalance of about 25% but potentially blinding, is cytomegalovirus infection of the retina. The fundus picture, with white retinal opacification surrounded by haemorrhage – described as 'cottage cheese and ketchup' – is striking.

Treatment is a matter for the specialist. Severe infections by *Toxoplasma gondii*, herpes simplex or herpes zoster, with their characteristic ophthalmic manifestations, are frequently seen in advanced stages of AIDS.

Other inflammatory disorders

Other inflammatory disorders of the choroid and retina are considered in Chapter 7.

10
Trauma

Blunt injury

Without rupture of the globe

Blunt injuries are caused by fists, blows during sport and a multitude of domestic and industrial mishaps. The effects range from a simple 'black eye' to gross disorganization of the globe:

1. The cornea may be abraded (see p. 56).
2. Conjunctival lacerations merit referral, because of the possibility of a concealed rupture of the globe.
3. Subconjunctival haemorrhage needs no treatment, provided vision is unimpaired.
4. Blood in the anterior chamber (hyphaema) shows as diffuse cloudiness of the aqueous, obscuring details of the iris and of the deeper parts of the eye. The blood settles in the lowest part, where it lies with a characteristic fluid level (Figure 10.1). Sometimes the anterior chamber becomes filled with blood. Referral is advised.
5. Traumatic mydriasis: persistent dilatation of the pupil due to damage of the iris sphincter is a common result of contusion, and if sufficiently severe may affect accommodation. It generally recovers. Alternatively, the root of the iris may be torn (iridodialysis).
6. Traumatic cataract can follow contusion. In severe injuries, the lens is torn from its attachment, prolapsing forward through the pupil or falling back into the vitreous (subluxation or dislocation). The presence of gross visual defect indicates major damage.

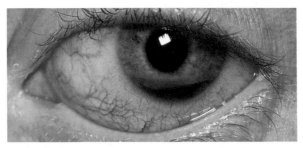

Fig. 10.1   Hyphaema: note slight eccentricity of pupil – traumatic mydriasis

7. In the posterior segment, there may be bleeding into the vitreous or damage to the retina. Retinal oedema (commotio retinae) shows as a greyish area in the fundus where detail is obscured and there may be small retinal haemorrhages. It usually resolves, though it is occasionally followed by pigmentary retinal changes and permanent visual loss.

8. The retina may be torn by the distortion of the eye at the time of the injury, leading to retinal detachment. This may be delayed for months or years. Treatment is surgical.

9. Choroidal tears are sometimes seen and appear as scars, concentric with the disc and close to the posterior pole. These represent areas of choroidal atrophy through which the white sclera is visible.

Rupture of the globe

Sometimes the coats of the eye are not able to resist the pressure at the moment of impact, and rupture occurs, most commonly at the junction of cornea and sclera. There will be haemorrhage within the eye. Examination will show the rupture and there will usually be ocular contents presenting in the wound. Vision is grossly impaired and these injuries are unlikely to be missed unless lid swelling prevents adequate examination. Some attempt must always be made to examine the eye and to assess visual acuity. Defective vision, as in any eye problem, is the finding most likely to indicate the possibility of serious trouble.

Penetrating injuries

Without retention of a foreign body

Potential causes include scissors, arrows, darts, flying particles (particularly in industry) and fragments of windscreens. The resultant injury is usually severe, though penetration by such things as fine wire can be difficult to see.

There will be a history of something having struck the eye, which will be photophobic and watering, with impaired vision. If the wound is in the anterior part of the eye, the pupil is usually distorted and there may be prolapse of the iris through the wound (Figure 10.2). Examination of the deeper eye is difficult on account of photophobia and haziness of the ocular structures. The lens may become opaque.

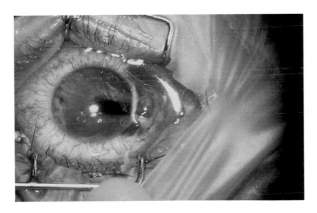

Fig. 10.2   Penetrating wound: note iris prolapse through open wound

In a child, examination of the injured eye is particularly difficult. A child is sometimes loath to admit that he/she has sustained an injury. It may not be until the eye becomes red and painful during the subsequent days that the true position becomes apparent.

Treatment of these wounds is surgical, with wound cleansing and repair under general anaesthesia. The prognosis for vision must be guarded.

With retention of a foreign body

These injuries are almost always industrial. Although provided with goggles, workers often fail to protect themselves adequately. The commonest cause of penetrating eye injuries is the hammer, striking a chisel or other metal tool. This throws off a steel flake which travels at high speed and penetrates the eye. These flakes are usually sterile and enter the eye through a small wound. The worker may scarcely notice the incident, subsequently complaining simply that he got 'something in his eye'. This makes diagnosis difficult, and demands constant awareness of the possibility of a penetrating injury if the foreign body is not visibly embedded in the surface of the cornea. A piece of steel in the eye will, in the course of months or years, induce a chronic chemical reaction and may ultimately destroy sight (siderosis bulbi).

Examination may show a wound of entry; with prolapse of the iris this is not likely to be mistaken. Difficulty arises if the entry wound is small, perhaps lying at the margin of the cornea, or in the sclera where it is covered by conjunctiva. A localized subconjunctival haemorrhage is a danger sign. The cornea must be stained with fluorescein and the eye examined in a good light. Even if the entry wound is not visible, a hole in the substance of the

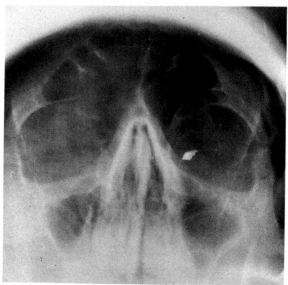

Fig. 10.3   Radiograph showing metallic intraocular foreign body

iris is diagnostic of a foreign body retained within the eye. The only sure diagnosis is by radiography (Figure 10.3), a routine in every case where the presence of an intraocular foreign body is suspected.

Treatment involves repair of the wound and removal of the foreign body after localization using X-rays. Removal may be by magnet if the particle is of steel, or by vitrectomy.

Sympathetic ophthalmitis

This rare condition may follow a penetrating injury of the eye. Persistent inflammation in the injured eye leads to low-grade irido-cyclitis in the fellow eye after 2 or 3 weeks or longer. This can be very destructive and difficult to control. The cause of the condition is poorly understood, but it represents a sensitivity reaction in the second eye. The decision as to whether or not an injured eye should be removed, in the face of a possible risk to the other eye, can be difficult.

Injuries to the orbit

Orbital haematoma may follow contusion, and fracture of the orbital bones may displace or damage the extraocular muscles.

Double vision suggests the possibility of a 'blow-out' fracture (Figure 10.4), and all contusion injuries leading to double vision should be referred. In 'blow-out' fracture an extraocular muscle becomes trapped in a fracture of the floor or, occasionally, the medial wall of the orbit. There is enophthalmos, due to prolapse of the orbital contents, and limitation of movement, usually on upward gaze.

The X-ray finding of a 'tear-drop' opacity in the antrum (Figure 10.5) is characteristic of a 'blow-out' fracture of the orbital floor. The orbit may have to be explored to free the trapped muscle and cover the bony defect.

Occasionally a blow to the head may interfere with the delicate blood supply of the optic nerve as it passes through the optic canal, causing severe visual impairment in the affected eye. Optic nerve damage is indicated by an afferent pupillary defect. Optic atrophy appears after a few weeks. Early decompression of the optic nerve is sometimes undertaken. A squint, usually divergent, may develop later.

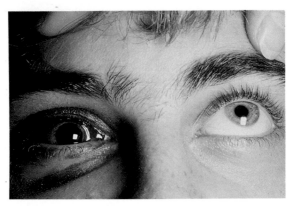

Fig. 10.4 'Blow-out' fracture: note failure of right eye to elevate on upward gaze (pupil dilated due to mydriatic drops)

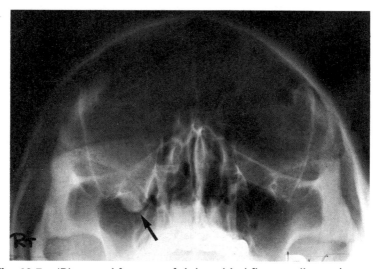

Fig. 10.5 'Blow-out' fracture of right orbital floor: radiograph shows 'tear-drop' opacity in antrum

Non-accidental injury in children

Bruising, usually of the face, thorax or buttocks is a cardinal sign, but up to 40% of non-accidentally injured children have eye injuries.

Retinal haemorrhage, which may be associated with intracranial bleeding and thoracic compression, is a cardinal sign – though there are many other possible causes of this condition. Also commonly seen as non-accidental injuries are subconjunctival haemorrhage and periorbital oedema. Any injury of the eye or visual pathway is a possibility, but haemorrhage within the optic canal, caused by shearing forces associated with vigorous shaking of the child, is a frequent finding. Such haemorrhage may lead to optic nerve infarction, with a blind eye and non-reacting pupil; when found at post mortem, it is said to be diagnostic of non-accidental injury.

11
Refractive errors

The formation of a clearly focused retinal image depends on the presence of a normal relationship between the axial length of the eye and the focal length of the lens system. The term 'lens system' is used because there are two elements involved in the refraction of light entering the eye. One is the biconvex lens and the other, more powerful from the optical point of view, the convex anterior surface of the cornea – where up to two-thirds of the refraction actually occurs.

Accommodation

If the eye is to achieve a clear image of objects at varying distances, it must adapt the focal length of the lens system to suit the varying angle of entry of rays of light. This is achieved by changing the curvature of the lens – accommodation.

The lens consists of a transparent mass of lens matter enclosed in an elastic membrane, the lens capsule. The lens is supported within the circle of the ciliary body by a series of fine fibres – the zonule, or suspensory ligament. The ciliary body contains a mass of muscle fibres innervated by the parasympathetic element of the third cranial nerve. By contraction, it can alter the tension in the suspensory ligament and thus in the lens capsule. Contraction of the ciliary muscle increases the curvature of the lens, and so shortens its focal length.

The stimulus for accommodation is reflex, based on the need to maintain a clear retinal image (Figure 11.1). There is a natural

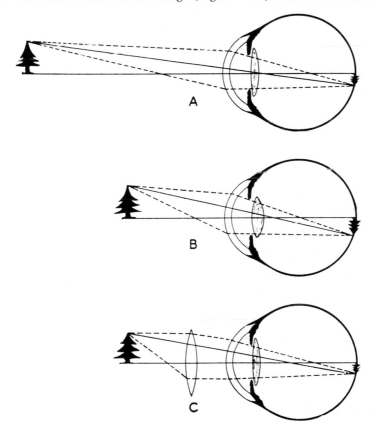

Fig. 11.1   Formation of the retinal image: (A): in the normal eye, with the accommodation relaxed, the image of a distant object falls on the retina; (B): when the object approaches the eye, a change of shape of the lens occurs and the image remains focused on the retina – this is accommodation; (C): with increasing age, the eye loses its power to change its focus to accommodate close objects, and has to be reinforced by a convex lens to keep the image in focus – this is presbyopia

relationship between the accommodative effort needed to produce a clear retinal image, and the amount of convergence of the visual axes needed to keep the images on the fovea of both eyes. The importance of the balance between these two functions is considered below in the discussion of errors of refraction in relation to the aetiology of squint (AC/A ratio).

Presbyopia

With increasing age, the lens of the eye becomes larger and less able to respond to the efforts of the ciliary body to alter its curvature. At about 45 years of age, close work such as reading and sewing becomes more difficult and by 65 years of age all power of accommodation is lost. The middle-aged must simply accept the need to wear glasses for close work. Whether these are bifocal, varifocal or simple reading glasses is purely a matter of choice.

Hyperopia (hypermetropia, long sight)

This is the commonest refractive error. Almost universal in infants, it lessens during the growing years, a process known as emmetropization. An exception to this regulatory mechanism occurs in Down's syndrome. These children tend to develop increasing, rather than decreasing, refractive errors due to defective coordination of the growth of the various refractive components of the eye – corneal curvature, lens form and axial length. The exact cause is unknown.

In hyperopia, when the accommodation is relaxed, rays of light from an object in the distance are brought to a focus behind the retina (Figure 11.2). In youth, if the degree of hyperopia is slight, this defect is of no disadvantage as it can be overcome by accommodation – but reading may demand effort.

Hyperopia needs correction only if it cannot be overcome comfortably by the eye's own focusing mechanism. It should, however, be corrected in children with amblyopia of one eye, or with convergent squint due to unequal refractive errors.

A degree of hyperopia insufficient to cause symptoms in youth may, with the natural lessening of the power of accommodation, give rise to reading difficulties in middle life. There will be an earlier demand for reading glasses from hyperopic patients than in those with no refractive error (emmetropic).

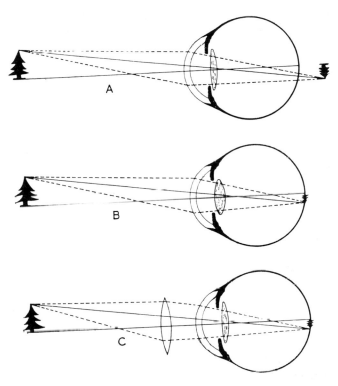

Fig. 11.2 Hyperopia: (A): with the accommodation relaxed, the image of a distant object falls behind the retina; (B): an effort of accommodation is needed for the clear viewing of an object, even in the distance; (C): this effort has to increase as the object becomes closer – if the error cannot comfortably be overcome by accommodation, a convex spectacle will be needed

Myopia (short sight)

In myopia, rays of light from a distant object are focused in front of the retina, either because the eye is excessively long or the refractive elements – cornea and lens – too powerful to produce a clearly focused image on distance fixation (Figure 11.3). Myopes are at a disadvantage compared to hyperopes in that they are unable to obtain clear distance vision by the exercise of accommodation. At close range, however, the advantage is with the myopes, who can focus on near objects with little or no effort of accommodation.

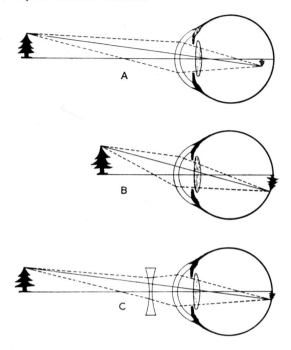

Fig. 11.3 Myopia: (A): the image of a distant object falls in front of the retina, and effort of accommodation will only increase the blurring; (B): near objects are clearly seen with little or no accommodation; (C): for clear distance sight, concave glasses are needed

Myopia is of two types: simple myopia, which is common; and progressive or degenerative myopia, which is uncommon.

Simple myopia

Simple myopia is often hereditary. With growth, the globe becomes too long. The onset is usually at about puberty, hence the term 'school short sight', but it may be delayed into early adult life.

The system of routine examination of schoolchildren generally leads to prompt recognition of the condition. Alternatively, the teacher notices that the child is not able to see teaching aids from the back of the classroom. In the case of preschool children, parents complain that the child holds books very close to his/her face, or sits too near the television.

Simple myopia advances during the school years and the need for new glasses can only be determined by regular examination. The child can lead a normal life and can play most games in splinter-proof glasses or contact lenses. It is not essential that glasses be worn from morning to night, but they should be worn in class and at other times when clear distance vision is required. As the child grow older, he/she will decide independently when glasses are to be worn.

Particular attention should be paid to the vision of siblings when there is a short-sighted child in the family.

Measures to arrest or prevent myopia, apart from refractive surgery, have failed to gain general acceptance.

Retinal detachment is more common in myopes than in normal-sighted individuals, the incidence increasing with the degree of myopia.

Degenerative myopia

This is a condition of unknown cause, associated with a very high degree of myopia and with pathological changes within the eye. Among these are vitreous opacities, cataract formation and degenerative changes at the posterior pole of the eye, often leading to the destruction of central vision (Figure 9.5).

Astigmatism

Astigmatism is usually due to the curvature of the cornea not being the same in all meridians. It may be associated with either hyperopia or myopia, and a cylindrical lens is needed to correct it. Failure to correct higher degrees of astigmatism during the years of visual development may lead to partial amblyopia.

There are some pathological conditions which, by causing distortion of the cornea, produce irregular astigmatism. Among these are diseases of the cornea such as keratoconus, corneal ulceration of various types, tarsal cysts, and the results of injury.

Ocular headache

Headache is a very common complaint, and it is certainly prominent among the reasons for which patients are referred for an ophthalmic opinion.

The ocular headache is often related to, or precipitated by, the use of the eyes. Thus it occurs on prolonged reading or sewing, watching television, or taking up a clerical occupation for the first time. The pain may be delayed in onset, appearing in the morning after an evening of ocular activity. It may be felt in the eyes themselves, or in the temple or occiput, in which case it is probably coming from the neck muscles. Ocular headache is usually regular in occurrence. A pain appearing at long intervals, without any change of ocular habit, is not likely to be of ocular origin. The same can be said of a pain of recent onset, when there has been no change in the use of the eyes.

Sufferers of migraine often present with ocular symptoms such as flickering lights and hemianopia (see Figures 14.8 and 14.9), but the headache which follows is unlikely to be influenced by glasses.

Refractive changes in diabetes

About a third of diabetics, particularly those with high levels of blood glucose, show a temporary change towards myopia at the onset of the illness. This can precede other symptoms by several weeks or months. Patients in the presbyopic age group may find their reading glasses unnecessary but their distance vision blurred. An unexpected myopic shift in refraction should suggest the possibility of diabetes and the urine or blood should be tested for glucose level.

Transient hyperopia frequently occurs as the blood sugar level falls on starting treatment for diabetes. Glasses should not be prescribed until the condition has been stable for several weeks.

Contact lenses

Contact lenses may be used as an alternative to spectacles for the correction of all refractive efforts. In general, the greater the refractive error, the greater the relative benefit from contact lenses. However, cosmetic reasons and the advantages of unobstructed vision cause many patients to prefer contact lenses to spectacles. Occasionally contact lenses are ordered as part of the treatment of eye disorders rather than on purely optical grounds – for example, in keratoconus where the astigmatism is too great to be corrected by spectacles, and in some cases of corneal ulceration, for protective purposes.

Contact lenses are of two main types, according to the material from which they are made: rigid and soft (hydrophilic).

Rigid lenses

Rigid ('hard') lenses are made of one of a variety of materials. Perspex, the standard for many years, has been overtaken in popularity by newer substances with less tendency to deprive the cornea of oxygen. Hypoxia leads to fluid retention within the corneal stroma and oedema of the epithelium, which leads to discomfort and blurred vision.

Rigid lenses have to be fitted so as to minimize oxygen deprivation and, in general, their wear must be restricted so that the oxygen supply of the cornea can be replenished. The commonest problems presented to the doctor by wearers of rigid contact lenses are associated with oxygen deprivation, usually caused by wearing the lenses too long, and minor trauma caused by their insertion or removal. Patients with problems associated with contact lens wear should be advised not to use the lens for 48 hours. The wearing-time should then be extended gradually, in the way most patients are advised when beginning to use lenses.

Infection is also a potential danger, though less so than with soft lenses. The spectrum of damage extends from small, sterile corneal infiltrates consisting of aggregations of leucocytes, to severe, suppurative infection. The cleaning of both the lenses and their container is important.

An apparently lost contact lens may sometimes be found in the superior conjunctival fornix on everting the upper lid (see Figure 5.1).

Women taking oral contraceptives may have slightly impaired tolerance of contact lens wear.

Soft lenses

Soft, or hydrophilic, lenses conform to the curvature of the cornea and are classified according to the material of which they are made and to their water content, which may range from 40 to 90%. The materials of higher water content tend to permit more diffusion of oxygen through the lens to the cornea. The lenses must always be kept in an appropriate storage solution. If allowed to dry they become distorted and brittle, and cannot be used until fully rehydrated.

Soft lenses are more widely used than the rigid type, and they have the advantages of longer initial wearing-times and greater initial comfort. They produce less distortion of the cornea in use, so may be more readily interchanged with spectacles, allowing intermittent use, for example in sport. Soft lenses are larger than the rigid type, usually overlapping the cornea by 1–2 mm. Certain soft lens materials allow extended wear for days, weeks, or even months. Those intended only for daily wear should be removed before sleep.

Sterility is of great importance with soft contact lenses, as the material from which they are made can become contaminated by bacteria or by *Acanthamoeba* (see p. 63). Care has to be taken when handling the lenses, and the user should wash his/her hands before inserting or removing a lens. The lens is generally rubbed with a surface cleaning agent after removal from the eye, and disinfected with chemicals or by heat. Soft lenses attract protein deposits, which are usually removed weekly by enzyme tablets.

Extended-wear lenses carry the greatest risk of infection. Any infection is potentially serious, and may lead to corneal ulceration and irreversible vascularization. Should infection be suspected, lens wear must be discontinued and appropriate antibiotic treatment instituted. The cornea must be checked by slit-lamp examination before lens wear is resumed.

It is with disinfecting agents containing thiomersal that problems with soft contact lenses are most frequently associated. These agents are toxic in high concentrations, and accumulate in the contact lens. The symptoms of toxic effects of lens disinfectants are lens intolerance and discomfort. The signs are red eye, with hyperaemia and hypertrophy of the conjunctival papillae (Figure 11.4). A soft lens wearer who becomes intolerant of disinfecting chemicals is usually advised to change to boiling the lenses in normal saline without preservative, or to clean them in hydrogen peroxide. An alternative is to use soft lenses which are discarded after a single day's use, so no preservatives or cleaning agents are required. These lenses are, however, expensive.

Infection, with corneal ulceration, is a less common but serious problem. Ulceration can lead to corneal vascularization. Should this occur, soft lens wear must be discontinued until the ulcer has healed and all new vessels have regressed. Antibiotic drops are prescribed. Gradually increasing vascularization from the corneal periphery may also occur without infection, probably in response to hypoxia. Hence soft lens wearers should have a periodic slit-

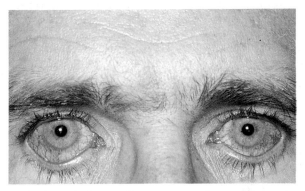

Fig. 11.4   Conjunctivitis medicamentosa, due to contact lens soaking-solution

lamp examination.

Soft lenses give less satisfactory visual acuity than rigid lenses if used to correct refractive errors which include significant degrees of astigmatism. They are also less durable and have to be discarded if damaged, discoloured or affected by protein deposition.

Technique for removal of a contact lens (Figure 11.5)

A GP may occasionally be called upon to remove a contact lens from an eye which is irritable or inflamed, for example in an elderly patient who has been fitted with an extended-wear soft lens and is unable to get to the specialist. The technique is:

1. Open the eye widely, with the index fingers behind the lashes of each lid.
2. Gently press the lid margins together so that they touch the edges of the contact lens. This will release the lens from the surface of the eye. It can then be picked off the lid margin.
3. If the first attempt is not successful, try again.

Tear production

Inadequate tear secretion is often a cause of poor tolerance of contact lenses of any type. Tear production can be assessed by Schirmer's test (Figure 4.2).

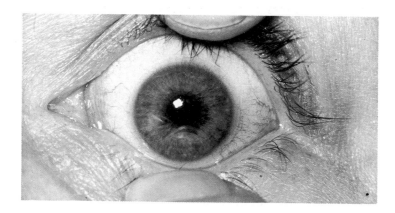

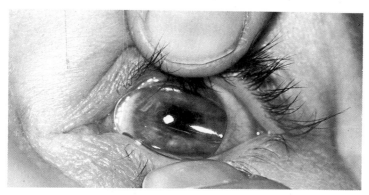

Fig. 11.5   Removal of soft contact lens

Drugs and contact lenses

Printed on the packets of some eye drop preparations are the words: 'not to be used with contact lenses'. This is a controversial matter, and it applies particularly to soft lenses. There are two possible reasons for advising against the use of certain eye drops with contact lenses:

1. The drops may, in the long term, damage or discolour the contact lens.
2. The drops contain a preservative, commonly benzalkonium chloride or thiomersal, to which the lens wearer may develop an adverse local reaction.

However, lens preservation intolerance develops in only a few cases, and usually after at least 6 months' use. So on neither count need the manufacturer's advice be taken too seriously if the eye drops must be used and the patient insists on wearing the lenses.

It is of greater importance that a contact lens is not worn when there is an eye disorder, such as keratitis or conjunctivitis, in which the lens might be implicated. 'When in doubt, take it out' is sound advice for any contact lens wearer.

Refractive surgery

Patients may seek the GP's advice on this subject. Refractive surgery does not address the more fundamental problems associated with the elongated, myopic eye – particularly degeneration of the central retina, leading to myopic macular degeneration, and of the peripheral retina, leading to retinal detachment. The surgery is solely directed at the refractive error. It must also be remembered that a myope who undergoes surgery to eliminate his refractive error will require reading glasses, as would an emmetrope, on reaching the age of presbyopia.

Corneal procedures

Permanent alteration of the refractive state of the eye by safe and predictable surgery has proved an elusive goal for ophthalmologists. It is not recommended for patients below the age of 21 years. Surgery to correct hyperopia has yet to gain wide acceptance. Indications in myopia include: intolerance of contact lenses combined with a dislike of, or fear of losing, glasses; a desire to improve unaided visual acuity for occupational reasons; or to make possible participation in outdoor sports such as skiing and mountaineering without optical aids. There are two currently-used procedures which are appropriate for treating myopia of up to about –6 dioptres – excimer laser photo-refractive keratectomy (PRK) and radial keratotomy (RK). In cases of myopia of up to –6 dioptres the results of both procedures are good, but with greater refractive errors they are less predictable. Excimer laser PRK is likely eventually to supersede RK, but the two techniques give comparable results.

Excimer laser photo-refractive keratectomy (PRK) (Figures 11.6a and 11.6b)

After careful preoperative evaluation and counselling, the epithelium of the cornea is removed surgically under topical anaesthesia, and the patient is instructed to look at the fixation light on the laser, so that the central optical zone is treated. The procedure lasts about 30 seconds, during which repeated laser pulses sculpt away the apical tissue of the cornea in a manner determined by the computer within the instrument. It takes 2 days for the epithelium to become re-established, and a further 2 or 3 weeks for the refraction to stabilize; there is usually an initial over-correction.

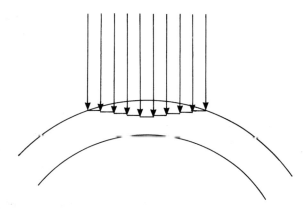

Fig. 11.6a Excimer laser photorefractive keratectomy, sectional view showing laser sculpting of central optical zone

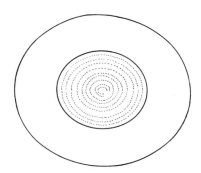

Fig. 11.6b Excimer laser photorefractive keratectomy, surface view

For lower degrees of myopia the results are excellent, but the higher the refractive error – and, paradoxically, the greater the patient's need for the procedure – the less predictable is the outcome. Principal complications are inaccuracies in correction and corneal scarring: the latter usually diminishes within 6 to 12 months, but may impair acuity while it persists.

Radial keratotomy (RK) (Figures 11.7a and 11.7b)

This is a procedure in which four or more radial incisions are made in the corneal periphery, leaving the central optical zone untouched and resulting in corneal flattening. Disadvantages of this procedure are an uncommon but worrying tendency to develop late refractive drift towards hyperopia, and weakening of the cornea, putting its integrity at risk in the event of a severe contusion injury.

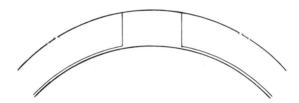

Fig. 11.7a   Radial keratotomy, sectional view: preset diamond blade incises cornea to about 95% depth, sparing central optical zone

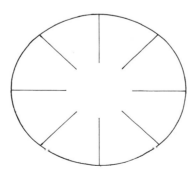

Fig. 11.7b   Radial keratotomy, surface view

Surgery for higher myopia

Above –6 dioptres, surgical treatment is more controversial unless the intention is to reduce, rather than eliminate, the refractive error. Excimer laser PRK has proved disappointing, but a variant, LASIK (laser in situ keratomileusis), shows great promise – though it is a complex procedure. A suction ring is applied to the eye to elevate the intraocular pressure temporarily, and a flap of superficial cornea is created with an automated micro-keratome, similar to a mechanized wood-plane. The underlying corneal stroma is then treated with excimer laser in a manner similar to that in surface PRK, and the flap of superficial cornea is replaced. Suturing is unnecessary. Early reports of the results are very promising, but the technique has yet to gain wide acceptance.

Non-corneal procedures

For high myopes who are intolerant of spectacles and contact lenses, an anterior chamber lens implant of negative power, can be inserted without lens extraction. The early visual results are excellent but longer-term complications remain uncertain, particularly with regard to the possibility of progressive corneal changes leading to decompensation and oedema, perhaps years later.

Clear lens extraction is another procedure which has been tried. The principal disadvantage is an increased incidence of retinal detachment, to which the myope is already prone. As in the case of negative power implants, clear lens extraction has not gained wide acceptance.

If cataract develops in later life, the elimination of either myopia or hyperopia by the appropriate selection of lens implant power is straightforward.

12
Ocular motility

Squint (strabismus)

A squint is present when the image of an object falls on the fovea of one eye but not that of the other. Squints may be classified as:

1. Concomitant (or non-paralytic). The angle of deviation does not vary with the direction of gaze.
2. Paralytic. The angle of deviation varies with the direction of gaze.

Concomitant squint

Development

The central part of the retina, the macula, is the only part with which detail can be seen, and an inborn reflex normally brings the image of an object onto the fovea. Normally the eyes are aligned in order to avoid double vision (diplopia). If any ocular disorder prevents the proper development of binocular vision, a squint may result.

The role of errors of refraction in the development of a squint is illustrated in Figure 12.1. To look at a close object, it is necessary not only to focus the eyes by the use of accommodation but also to exercise convergence. In hyperopia, the amount of accommodation is out of proportion to the amount of convergence needed at a given distance. The child may not be able to dissociate these functions, with resultant over-convergence.

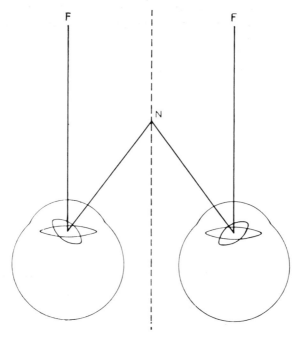

Fig. 12.1   The accommodation–convergence relationship: if the eyes are considered, in the first instance, as viewing a distant object (F), a clear retinal image is obtained in each eye without effort of either accommodation or convergence; on viewing a near object (N), a balanced relationship normally exists between the degree of accommodation exerted and the angle of convergence – in hyperopia, this relationship is upset

Causes

The main causes of concomitant squint in childhood are:
- Heredity
- High degrees of refractive error
- Ocular disease, preventing the proper development of vision
- Cerebral palsy, hydrocephalus and other neurological disorders
- Down's syndrome, Turner's syndrome and other causes of multiple handicap.

The onset of a squint in a predisposed child is often associated with some external event, such as a severe illness. It has been suggested that the reduction in incidence of concomitant convergent squint (see below) by about 50% over the period 1970–1990 may reflect the near-disappearance of measles due to widespread immunization.

Disease-related causes of squint are corneal opacities, cataract, retinal diseases and optic atrophy.

Classification

Concomitant squint may be classified as:
- convergent (esotropia)/divergent (exotropia)
- Constant/intermittent
- Uniocular/alternating.

Convergent squint (esotropia)

Presentation

Although occasionally present at birth, the onset of a convergent squint occurs typically at around 3 years of age. The deviation, intermittent at first, is often noticed by someone other than the parents, and is more obvious when the child is tired, angry or unwell.

A child does not 'grow out of' a squint, and time spent waiting for spontaneous cure is time wasted. Early referral is mandatory – firstly because intermittent squints may be controllable with glasses alone if they are treated early, and secondly because amblyopia, which usually accompanies a squint, is easier to treat the earlier the child presents.

Diagnosis

The commonest cause of a mistaken diagnosis of a squint is epicanthus, making the cornea seem closer to the midline than it actually is (Figure 12.2). If in any doubt, the relative positions of the bright reflexes from the cornea must be assessed. If the eyes are 'straight', the bright reflections of a torch will be symmetrical.

The other invaluable test for a squint is the cover test (Figure 12.3). With the child looking at an object, each eye is covered in turn. If the eye remains stationary when the fellow eye is covered, no squint is present. If, however, the eye moves to take up fixation when the fellow eye is covered, that eye was originally squinting.

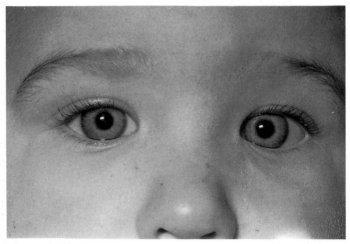

Fig. 12.2   Epicanthus: note symmetry of corneal light reflexes

Treatment

The treatment of squint consists of the following steps, the detailed application of which will be decided by the ophthalmologist:

1. *Refraction*, under the influence of a cycloplegic, fundus examination through the dilated pupil and the provision of spectacles if indicated (Figure 12.4).

2. *Occlusion of the fixing eye*, to force the amblyopic eye into activity.

3. *Orthoptic supervision*, to assess the state of binocular vision, monitor amblyopia treatment and assist in the planning of surgery.

4. *Operation* may be required in the treatment of those who do not respond to the provision of glasses together with orthoptic treatment. Adjustment of the visual axes is achieved by weakening (recession) of the overactive muscles, sometimes combined with strengthening (advancement or resection) of the antagonists. The extent of the surgery is largely based on measurements obtained in the Orthoptic Department. Adult squint surgery often makes use of the adjustable suture technique, where approximate ocular alignment is achieved by surgery under general anaesthesia. Following recovery and with orthoptic measurement and local anaesthesia, the knots are untied, and adjustment is carried out by either tightening or releasing the suture as required.

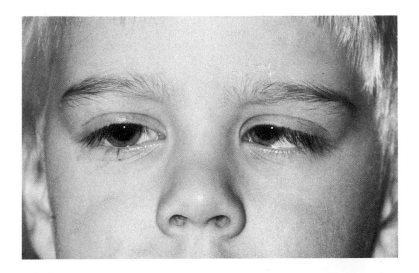

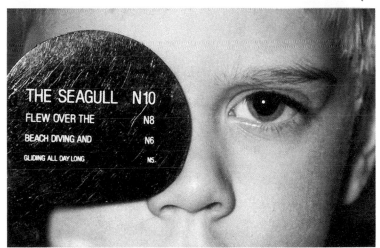

THE SEAGULL   N10
FLEW OVER THE   N8
BEACH DIVING AND   N6
GLIDING ALL DAY LONG   N5

Fig. 12.3   The cover test: left convergent squint

In cases with incurable amblyopia, when the problem is purely cosmetic, surgery is the only possible treatment. The hospital stay is short, and the patient will go home following full recovery from the anaesthetic.

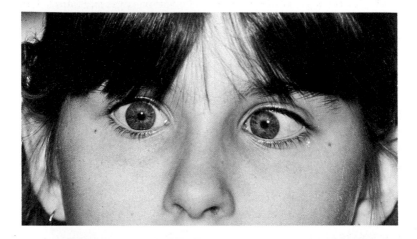

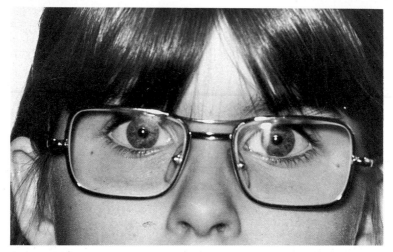

Fig. 12.4   Accommodative convergent squint, controlled with spectacles

Divergent squint (exotropia)

This condition is less common than convergent squint. It presents at a later age and is usually seen on distant gaze. The child may be noticed to close one eye in bright light. Divergent squint is less commonly associated with amblyopia than is convergent squint, but the child may by myopic.

Operation is generally advised if the squint is present more than 50% of the time or is cosmetically unsatisfactory. The prognosis is good. Older children with intermittent diplopia associated with a divergent squint may also require surgery.

Latent squint (heterophoria)

In adults, a state of imbalance between the muscles of the two eyes may not be sufficient to lead to actual squint, but can lead to symptoms of eye-strain, particularly on reading. A well-defined cause of this difficulty is 'convergence insufficiency'. As is the case in various types of heterophoria, convergence insufficiency often responds to exercises prescribed by an orthoptist.

Paralytic squint

The cause of paralytic squints usually lies within the central nervous system. Most such squints occur in the elderly, and are due to small arteriosclerotic lesions. Recovery usually takes place within a few weeks. Alternatively, paralytic squints may be due to trauma, intracranial vascular accidents, aneurysms, tumours or multiple sclerosis.

Symptoms

The only symptom is diplopia, often leading to giddiness and nausea, and usually worse in one direction of gaze.

Diagnosis

A marked squint may be obvious, or there may be evident limitation of movement of an eye. The need to investigate patients with paralytic squint of recent onset depends on their age and on whether there are other neurological abnormalities. Referral is always appropriate.

The analysis of paralytic squint is depicted in Figure 12.5. The patient is asked to follow the movement of an object in the various directions of gaze, and the position of maximum separation of the images is determined. The eyes are then covered in turn, demonstrating which image is furthest displaced. The 'furthest away' image belongs to the eye with the paralysed muscle.

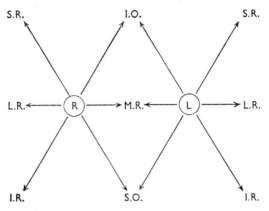

Fig. 12.5 Analysis of paralytic squint

Third nerve palsy: Complete oculomotor paralysis gives ptosis; a dilated, unreacting pupil with a normal consensual response in the other eye to a stimulus in the affected eye; and deviation of the paralysed eye laterally and downwards. This is due to the unopposed actions of the superior oblique and lateral rectus muscles. The acute onset of a third nerve palsy, associated with headache, may be due to an intracranial aneurysm and requires urgent referral to a neurosurgeon.

Usually, oculomotor nerve lesions are incomplete. A third nerve palsy sparing the pupil is likely to be due to arteriosclerosis or the vascular complications of diabetes. Recovery may be complicated by aberrant regeneration, leading to bizarre ocular movements.

Fourth nerve palsy: Trochlear nerve palsy is less common than lesions of the third and sixth nerves. Patients may adopt a compensatory head posture due to the vertical and torsional actions of the unopposed inferior oblique muscle. Their difficulty is in looking down and in reading. Bilateral superior oblique palsy is usually due to head injury.

Sixth nerve palsy: Weakness of the lateral rectus muscle produces defective abduction of the eye. The patient may adopt a head-turn toward the affected side to minimize diplopia.

Myasthenia gravis may present with ptosis (p. 30) or weakness of extraocular muscles leading to diplopia. Diagnosis is confirmed by a positive Tensilon® test and by the demonstration of motor endplate receptor antibodies in a blood sample.

Management

While a patient is awaiting recovery from an arteriosclerotic lesion, a temporary prism attached to the glasses, or an injection of botulinum toxin into the antagonist muscle, may be helpful. If recovery fails to occur, surgery may be indicated to restore an effective, if not a complete, field of binocular vision.

Patients with paralytic diplopia should not drive. A paralytic squint in an older, arteriosclerotic patient should be regarded as a minor stroke and may be the forerunner of a major cerebrovascular accident.

Gaze palsy

Interference with the supranuclear control of eye movements leads to limitation of gaze in one or more directions. The cause may be multiple sclerosis, Parkinson's disease, a vascular lesion or a tumour. A neurologist's advice should be sought.

Internuclear ophthalmoplegia

Failure of either eye to adduct on lateral gaze, with nystagmus of the abducting eye, is due to a lesion in the medial longitudinal bundle. Internuclear ophthalmoplegia is common in multiple sclerosis: in the elderly it is usually due to a mid-brain stroke.

Nystagmus

Nystagmus – involuntary, oscillatory movements of the eyes – is either jerky, with fast and slow components, or pendular. The cause may be in the labyrinthine or visual systems.

Diagnosis

Jerky nystagmus is seen under certain circumstances in normal individuals. The induction of nystagmus on caloric stimulation of the ears and on rotation of the head is mediated via the vestibular system. Optokinetic nystagmus occurs when objects are fixated in rapid succession, as when looking through the window of a moving train. In 'end point' nystagmus the eyes oscillate on extreme lateral gaze.

Vestibular nystagmus occurs in disorders of the middle ear and its central connections, and of the cerebellum. The movements are jerky, with the fast component toward the side of the lesion.

Pendular nystagmus is seen in children whose vision has been markedly impaired in both eyes since birth, or becomes so during the first year or two of life. It arises because the normal fixation reflexes cannot become established.

Congenital nystagmus is a fairly common inherited condition. The movements are horizontal, vertical or rotatory. Usually there is one position of gaze in which they are least marked, and the patient may adopt a compensatory head posture so that the eyes assume this position, thereby obtaining optimium vision. Corrective surgery or prismatic lenses sometimes help.

All cases of nystagmus should be referred. There may be underlying ocular disorders such as mild forms of albinism, but usually no treatment is available. Nystagmus with a vertical component is more likely to signify neurological disease; investigation with MRI or CT scanning is usually appropriate.

Management

In the absence of other ocular disorders, most children with congenital nystagmus achieve good near vision, so they can read small print and cope with normal schooling, but their distance vision is generally not better than 6/18 (Snellen). Hence parents should be warned that their child may not have good enough vision to be eligible for a driving licence (Ch. 18). This may have important consequences for employment.

Latent nystagmus

Latent nystagmus is not apparent when both eyes are fixing, but becomes manifest when either eye is covered. The condition is of no importance clinically unless the sight in one eye is lost, but it may be the cause of poor recorded acuity when each eye is tested separately. When tested with both eyes in use, vision is normal.

Amblyopia (lazy eye)

Amblyopia is defined as reduced acuity in an eye after correction of any refractive error, without detectable disorder of the ocular media, retina or visual pathways.

Ambylopia may be due to squint, particularly in children. Any misalignment, or obstacle, may prevent the binocular use of the eyes, and the child will disregard the image seen by one eye and concentrate on the other. This neglect of one eye can lead to the development of amblyopia. If allowed to persist beyond the age of about 7 years, the amblyopia will be irreversible and the vision will be permanently impaired.

Amblyopia may be caused by stimulus deprivation, as in ptosis or congenital cataract, in which the defect must be corrected as early as possible if useful vision is to be achieved.

If there are unequal refractive errors in the two eyes (anisometropia), amblyopia may result. A difference in hyperopia of >1 dioptre, or in myopia of >3 dioptres, may lead to ambylopia but not to a squint. Provided the refractive difference is not excessive, optical correction (sometimes combined with occlusion of the eye with normal vision) usually gives markedly improved, if not normal, acuity in the amblyopic eye. Best results are obtained in children under 6 or 7 years of age, but limited improvement may be obtained in older children.

Inadequately corrected astigmatism may lead to partial amblyopia in both eyes (meridional amblyopia).

Slight amblyopia, with reduced acuity when measured by reading Snellen test type lines, may escape detection with single letter matching tests like the Sheridan Gardiner (p. 8). This phenomenon, known as 'crowding', should be borne in mind when interpreting the results of letter matching tests.

13
Glaucoma

Any condition in which intraocular pressure is raised, with damage to vision, is glaucoma. An intraocular pressure of 21 mmHg is considered to be the upper limit of normal. However, about a fifth of cases of open-angle glaucoma have some features of the condition but pressure at or below 21 mmHg.

Aqueous is produced by the ciliary body and passes through the pupil to the anterior chamber. It leaves the chamber through pores in the trabecular meshwork, and enters the canal of Schlemm, an encircling channel at the corneoscleral junction. The aqueous returns to the blood stream via the episcleral plexus of veins.

Glaucoma is classified according its cause, and may be primary or secondary.

Primary glaucomas include:
  Congenital (buphthalmos)
  Primary angle-closure
  Primary open-angle (chronic simple)

Secondary glaucomas include:
  Pigmentary
  Pseudo-exfoliative
  Uveitic
  Lens-induced
  Post-traumatic
  Neovascular (thrombotic or diabetic)
  Steroid-induced
  All suspected cases of glaucoma should be referred, indicating priority.

Congenital glaucoma (buphthalmos)

Occasionally present at birth, this condition is so rare that a GP is unlikely to see it. Early recognition is essential for successful treatment.

In buphthalmos, congenital abnormalities in the trabecular meshwork impede the drainage of aqueous. The infant's eyes water profusely and are red and painful. Attacks of pain may be intermittent in the early stages. The cornea has a ground-glass appearance, and becomes enlarged beyond the normal diameter of 10.5 mm. There may be splits in the deeper layers of the cornea. The globe enlarges and the optic disc becomes cupped. Any suspected case must be referred urgently. Treatment is surgical.

Primary angle-closure glaucoma (acute or congestive glaucoma)

Acute glaucoma is one of the emergencies of ophthalmology; it is rare below the age of 60 years. A GP is unlikely to see more than one acute case in his lifetime. Gradual shallowing of the anterior chamber as the lens enlarges with age predisposes to angle-closure glaucoma; it cannot develop in eyes with deep anterior chambers (Figure 13.1).

The intraocular pressure rises, usually suddenly. The pupil becomes fixed in mid-dilatation and, with increasing pressure, corneal oedema occurs. The condition may also develop insidiously. Such cases are differentiated from open-angle glaucoma by detailed examination of the anterior chamber angle with a special contact lens (gonioscopy).

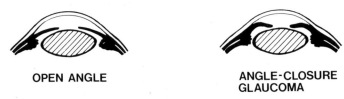

OPEN ANGLE   ANGLE-CLOSURE
                             GLAUCOMA

Fig. 13.1   Diagram of open and narrow angles

The use of mydriatic drops to dilate the pupil for examination of the fundus, for example in the routine review of diabetics, may, very rarely, precipitate an attack of angle-closure glaucoma. In eyes seen to have shallow anterior chambers, demonstrable by shining a light obliquely on to the cornea and finding only part of the convex iris illuminated, mydriatic drops should be used with caution. However, should an episode of acute angle-closure glaucoma occur in a controlled environment such as a diabetic clinic, it should be pointed out that such a situation would probably have occurred anyway at some time, and it is better for it to have done so where doctors are immediately available.

Presentation

Typically, the patient complains of sudden onset of pain with blurred vision (usually down to 'counting fingers' or 'hand movements'). Only one eye is affected, but the stress resulting from the attack may precipitate a similar situation in the other eye. Collapse and vomiting may occur if the pain is severe.

The eye is red, with corneal oedema preventing a clear view of iris detail, and the pupil is fixed and semidilated (Figure 13.2). Raised intraocular pressure is obvious on palpation of the eye through the closed lids; the eye feels stony-hard.

There may be a history of previous visual disturbance, particularly of seeing coloured haloes round white lights in the evening, perhaps with pain and blurring. These attacks may initially be self-limiting and relieved by sleep, during which the pupil normally contracts. Such a history requires referral as a glaucoma suspect, even without evidence of established angle-closure glaucoma.

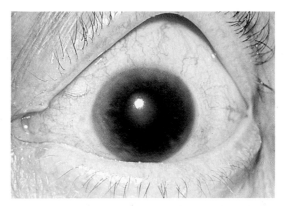

Fig. 13.2   Acute glaucoma: note hazy cornea and vertically-oval semidilated pupil

Management

All cases of angle-closure glaucoma must be referred as emergencies. Hospital treatment is with intravenous acetazolamide (Diamox®) 500 mg and oral acetazolamide 250 mg. Additional medical treatment may be necessary, and 2% pilocarpine is used prophylactically in the fellow eye. Definitive treatment is by YAG laser iridotomy – making one or more holes in the peripheral iris to permit the passage of aqueous into the anterior chamber, bypassing the pupil. Provided that permanent damage has not occurred in the drainage angle by adhesion formation, this procedure cures the patient. The fellow eye is usually given prophylactic iridotomy.

Primary open-angle glaucoma (chronic simple glaucoma)

A common and still incompletely understood condition, open-angle glaucoma occurs in about 2% of people over 40 years of age, with increasing incidence in older age groups. It is bilateral and a common cause of blindness: early diagnosis gives the best chance of satisfactory treatment. Family history is of great importance – the incidence in the children and siblings of glaucoma sufferers is several times higher than in the rest of the population. Under current (1997) UK legislation, individuals with a family history of this type of glaucoma are entitled to free eye tests by optometrists. Other risk factors in open-angle glaucoma have been identified as high myopia, ischaemic heart disease and a history of a bleeding episode requiring blood transfusion. Systemic hypertension is loosely associated with ocular hypertension and open-angle glaucoma.

Pathogenesis

Drainage of aqueous at the trabecular meshwork is impeded, despite free access to the angle, for reasons that are not clear. The consequence is raised intraocular pressure, resulting in damage to the disc. This leads to characteristic atrophy of the nerve fibres at the optic disc (cupping) (Figure 13.3) and visual field defects which, if the pressure is not controlled, may progress to blindness.

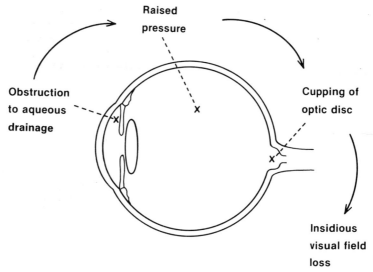

Fig. 13.3   Open-angle glaucoma

Diagnosis

Most cases are detected in the course of routine sight tests. Several surveys in the UK have shown that GPs had suspected the diagnosis in about 5% of patients referred to eye clinics and found to have glaucoma. The factors taken into account in making the diagnosis are:

- Cupping of the disc (see Figures 13.4a and 13.4b)
- Raised intraocular pressure
- Visual field (see Figures 13.5a and 13.5b).

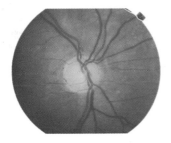

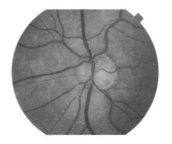

Fig. 13.4a Advanced glaucoma, 78-year-old female, right eye. Cup/disc ratio 0.9: note marked disc pallor

Fig. 13.4b Early glaucoma, left eye, same patient as in Figure 13.4a. Cup/disc ratio 0.4: note good disc colour and splinter haemorrhage at 4 o'clock within disc

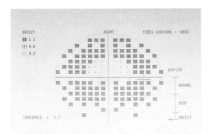

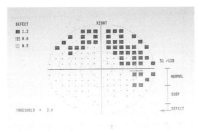

Fig. 13.5a Henson field chart of right eye of patient shown in Figures 13.4a and 13.4b, showing loss of peripheral field and preservation of central island

Fig. 13.5b Henson field chart of left eye of same patient as in Figure 13.5a, showing superior arcuate scotoma

Cupping of the disc

This is the feature most accessible to the GP, and every opportunity should be taken to practise the assessment of discs for possible glaucomatous changes. All doubtful cases, as well as those with apparently obvious changes, should be referred for further assessment. But identification is not easy; even experts find it impossible to distinguish normal from glaucomatous discs with certainty. The characteristics to look for in particular are the uniformity of width of the disc margin and symmetry in both eyes. Note should also be taken of:

1. *The size of the cup*, expressed as cup-disc ratio. 1.0 indicates complete cupping and 0.5 that the cup extends for half the overall disc diameter. 'Physiological' cupping is seen in healthy eyes, but a high cup-disc ratio carries a strong suspicion of glaucoma (see Figures 13.4a and 13.4b).

2. *A vertically oval cup* (vertical cup-disc ratio greater than horizontal ratio) is usually associated with glaucomatous field loss.

3. *Asymmetry* between the disc cupping in the two eyes suggests glaucoma.

4. *Haemorrhage* at the disc margin, suggesting circulatory embarrassment at the optic nerve head, makes a diagnosis of glaucoma likely to be correct.

5. *Pallor* of the disc is more difficult to evaluate: it may be of significance, but cupping is a more reliable sign. Advanced cases of glaucoma always have pale discs (see Figure 13.4a).

6. *Retinal vein occlusion*. Fundus examination showing extensive retinal haemorrhages due to retinal vein occlusion (Figures 9.4a and 9.4b) indicates immediate referral. A venous occlusion may be the presenting feature of glaucoma.

Raised intraocular pressure

There are as many pitfalls in intraocular pressure measurement and the conclusions drawn from it as there are from disc assessment. Guessing the pressure from palpation of the globe is useless, except in the extreme case of acute angle-closure glaucoma.

It is by no means incumbent on GPs to measure intraocular pressure (tonometry), but if a doctor or practice assistant is to do so, three suitable instruments are available. The Tonopen® is portable and simple to use (Figure 13.6). The Perkins hand-held applanation tonometer (Figure 13.7) is portable and accurate, but some practice is required to achieve proficiency in its use. More expensive, but rather easier to use, and of comparable accuracy, is the Keeler 'Pulsair®' tonometer (Figure 13.8). It has the advantage of being 'non-contact', so neither anaesthetic drops nor sterilization are required.

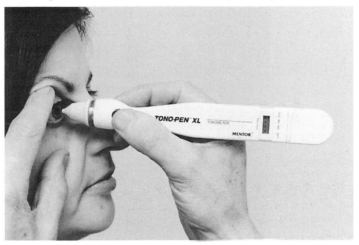

Fig. 13.6 Tonopen® tonometer

The increasing incidence of open-angle glaucoma over age 40 years makes tonometry a valuable screening procedure in routine medical checks. Tonometry is usually routinely carried out in the course of eye examination for refraction. Patients found at refraction to have intraocular pressures of >21 mmHg are commonly referred to their GP. It helps the ophthalmologist considerably if the referral letter is accompanied by all the details given on the report, together with relevant medical information, particularly with regard to respiratory and cardiovascular disorders.

It is common to find raised intraocular pressure without disc changes or field loss – termed 'ocular hypertension' (see below for management).

Visual field

To detect glaucomatous loss of visual field at an early stage is time-consuming and may require complex apparatus. This aspect of diagnosis is therefore outside the scope of general practice. Field

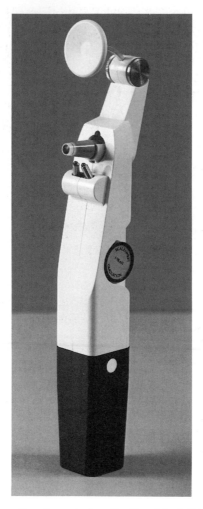

Fig. 13.7   Applanation tonometer: Perkins Mark 2 hand-held model

charts (Figures 13.5a and 13.5b) enclosed with letters from optometrists should be sent to the ophthalmologist with the referral letter.

Once field loss is significant enough to attract the patient's attention, the glaucoma is likely to be far advanced. Early diagnosis is the key to successful management.

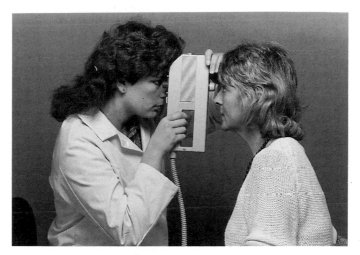

Fig. 13.8   Keeler 'Pulsair®' tonometer

Glaucomatous field loss tends to be more severe in patients with generalized arteriosclerosis, due, probably, to poor perfusion at the optic nerve head. Sudden exacerbation of field loss may be seen after acute illnesses such as coronary thrombosis, severe gastrointestinal haemorrhage or major surgery in which there has been a period of significantly lowered blood pressure.

Field loss and disc cupping without raised intraocular pressure represent damage to the disc without impaired drainage of aqueous. This condition is termed 'low-tension glaucoma'. Treatment is difficult.

Management

Suspected cases of open-angle glaucoma should be referred, indicating priority. It is preferable that treatment be withheld until after the first consultation with the specialist, so that a true baseline assessment can be made.

Raised pressure alone, without disc or field changes, ('ocular hypertension'), requires specialist follow-up but is not usually treated. Regular review of the condition is mandatory – monitoring of the state of the optic discs, and careful and repeated examination of the field of vision, should disclose changes promptly. If there is any evidence of change in the disc appearance or visual field loss, treatment for glaucoma must be given.

The choice of treatment for open-angle glaucoma is between drug therapy by eye drops (or, rarely, oral agents), conventional glaucoma drainage surgery and laser trabeculoplasty. It is usual to try drops initially. The other means are reserved for those who do not respond satisfactorily, due to either failure to tolerate the regime or its ineffectiveness – manifested by persistently raised pressure and progressive field loss. However, a growing body of ophthalmic opinion favours immediate laser trabeculoplasty or surgical trabeculectomy.

Glaucoma requires a lifetime of regular ophthalmic supervision, and the GP may be asked to make inquiries of defaulters. He/she also has a role in advising relatives of glaucoma patients, who are at risk, to seek appropriate examination.

Medical treatment

The drugs commonly used and their side-effects are listed in Table 13.1. Most frequently prescribed are topical beta-blockers and pilocarpine 0.5–4.0%. Pilocarpine is also available as slow-release inserts (Ocuserts®) which are placed in the conjunctival fornix and changed weekly. The GP should be aware of the potentially dangerous side-effects of beta-blockers. If in doubt, stop the drug and refer. Newer drugs than beta-blockers are useful when there are contraindications, such as asthma and cardiac disease.

Patient compliance is all-important, and it is the responsibility of the ophthalmologist, supported by the GP, to ensure that the patient understands why glaucoma drugs have been prescribed and that their aim is the preservation of useful sight, rather than the improvement of vision.

Surgical treatment

Patients in whom glaucoma is not adequately controlled by medical treatment require surgery to reduce the pressure. The target pressure is usually 21 mmHg, but it may be a considerably lower figure.

The surgical procedure most commonly use is trabeculectomy, in which a small block of tissue is removed from the trabecular mesh-work. A drainage 'bleb' or blister usually results and can be seen behind the limbus under the upper lid. The operation may be done under general or local anaesthesia. Accelerated cataract formation is a disadvantage of glaucoma surgery.

Table 13.1 Drugs commonly used in open-angle glaucoma

Group	Non-proprietary name	Proprietary name	Inconvenient side effects	Serious side effects
α_2-Adreno-ceptor agonists	Brimonidine tartrate 0.2% b.d.	Alphagan	Local allergy/irritation; dry mouth	
Beta-adrenergic antagonists (β-blockers)	Betaxolol 0.5% b.d.* Carteolol hydrochloride 1–2% b.d. Levobunolol hydrochloride 0.5% o.d. or b.d. Timolol maleate 0.25–0.5% b.d.	Betoptic Teoptic Betagan Timoptol	Local irritation	Bronchospasm; worsening of asthma and of chronic lung disease; hypotensive stroke; bradycardia Dangerous in heart block
Carbonic anhydrase inhibitors	Acetazolamide 0.5–2 G daily Acetazolamide 0.5–1G daily	Diamox Diamox SR	Gastro-intestinal disturbance; paraesthesiae	Blood dyscrasias; electrolyte disturbance; weight loss; urinary calculi
	Dorzolamide 2% t.i.d.	Trusopt	Local irritation; nausea; headache; malaise	Contraindicated in severe renal failure
Miotics (parasympathomimetics)	Pilocarpine 0.5–4% up to q.i.d.	Isotocarpine SNO-Pilo Pilo ocuserts	Brow ache; small pupils; transient myopia; gastro-intestinal spasm	
Prostaglandin analogues	Latanoprost 0.005% o.d.	Xalatan	Local irritation; increased iris pigmentation	
Sympatho-mimetics	Adrenaline 0.5–1% b.d. Dipivefrine hydrochloride 0.1% b.d.	Eppy Simplene Propine	Local irritation; red eyes; tachycardia	Angle-closure glaucoma with narrow angles; cystoid macular oedema in aphakia

Note *betaxolol is a cardio-selective β_1 antagonist and less likely to produce bronchoconstriction than the other β-blockers listed.

An alternative treatment is laser trabeculoplasty. Up to 100 small burns are applied by argon laser to the trabecular meshwork. This is an out-patient procedure without significant complications. It is successful in about 25% of cases for up to 5 years, making it particularly useful in the elderly.

Treatment by conventional drainage surgery or laser trabeculoplasty may free patients from the need to take regular medication, but most are advised to have periodic checks to ensure that the glaucoma remains satisfactorily controlled.

Secondary glaucomas

Pigmentary glaucoma

This is a bilateral disease, in which pigment is dispersed throughout the anterior segment of the eye. It usually occurs in males in the fourth or fifth decade. With the slit-lamp, pigment can be seen deposited on the corneal endothelium in a vertical line. Treatment is as for primary open-angle glaucoma, laser trabeculoplasty being most effective. Laser iridotomy also has a role.

Pseudo-exfoliative glaucoma

Pseudo-exfoliation syndrome (PXS) affects older patients: the cause is unknown. Whitish flakes of abnormal fibrillary material are deposited on the anterior lens surface, in the pupil margin and in the anterior chamber drainage angle. When PXS is associated with glaucoma, the response to medical treatment is poor and glaucoma surgery is often required. Cataract surgery is attended by a higher incidence of complications when PXS is present.

Uveitic glaucoma

Iritis or iridocyclitis may be accompanied by raised intraocular pressure, usually settling as the inflammation subsides. Drugs to reduce intraocular pressure may be needed in addition to those prescribed to control the uveitis (see p. 71).

Lens-induced glaucoma

A hypermature cataract, seen as a white opacity in the pupil, may degenerate and obstruct aqueous drainage by the collection of material in the trabeculum, or swell and cause angle-closure glaucoma. Any patient with a red painful eye and a dense, mature cataract should be referred urgently.

Post-traumatic glaucoma

Blunt injury, usually causing hyphaema (p. 69), may predispose to glaucoma by damaging the drainage angle. This accounts for a number of apparently unilateral cases of glaucoma. Patients who have sustained significant injury to an eye should be monitored with particular vigilance for glaucoma, and should report the history of injury when undergoing routine sight tests.

Neovascular (thrombotic or diabetic) glaucoma

This is associated with rubeosis iridis, common causes of which are central retinal vein occlusion with ischaemia, and proliferative diabetic retinopathy. Rubeosis iridis presents as pain in a blind eye (see p. 91). Onset occurs typically 3 months after the onset of central vein occlusion, though the interval may be much longer. New vessels are visible on the surface of the iris. The treatment of both neovascular glaucoma and rubeosis iridis is unsatisfactory.

Steroid-induced glaucoma

The use of steroid drops or ointment in or around the eye for periods longer than a week or two leads to raised intraocular pressure in susceptible individuals. Pressure checks are therefore necessary. If increased pressure is found and the continued use of steroid is considered essential, the ophthalmologist may decide to use one of the available steroids which are less likely to cause this side-effect, such as fluorometholone (FML®). The pressure returns to its previous level after stopping the steroid medication, but irreversible damage may have be done.

14
The visual pathway

Optic nerve
- Congenital abnormalities
- Optic atrophy
- Intrinsic tumours of the optic nerve

Papilloedema
Interference with visual pathway
Motor and sensory lesions
Migraine
Disorders of the pupil

Optic nerve

The GP can inspect the optic nerve at the optic disc, and can assess its function by testing pupil reactions, visual acuity, colour vision and visual fields. Complex equipment is needed to test function electrically (see Ch. 17).

Congenital abnormalities

A number of congenital abnormalities of the optic disc are recognized:
Myelinated nerve fibres (Figure 14.1)
Drusen of the optic disc (Figure 14.2)
Coloboma of the optic disc
Tilted optic disc
Optic disc hypoplasia
Optic disc pit.
Of these, drusen (hyaline-like, round deposits) may mimic papilloedema (see p. 164); coloboma and tilting of the optic disc may be associated with visual field defects. About 30% of eyes with optic disc pits later develop macular oedema and failure of central vision. Optic disc hypoplasia may be a cause of poor vision.

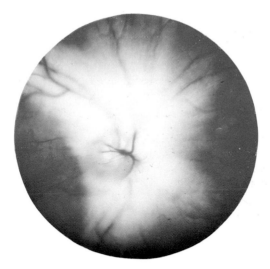

Fig. 14.1 Myelinated nerve fibres

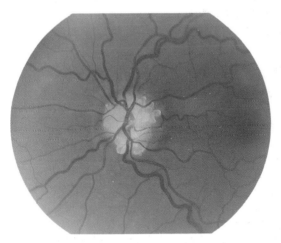

Fig. 14.2 Drusen of optic disc

Optic atrophy

Disorders of the optic nerve producing pallor of the optic disc (optic atrophy) are:

Trauma
Ischaemia of the retina
Ischaemia of the optic nerve
Optic neuritis
Compressive lesions of the visual pathway
Toxic or nutritional optic nerve damage
Glaucoma
Retinitis pigmentosa
Resolved papilloedema

Trauma

Usually, trauma is caused by a severe blow to the eye or side of the head. Apart from loss of vision, the only sign may be an afferent pupillary defect. Radiographs of the skull are advisable, but may show no fracture. Optic atrophy develops in 6–8 weeks.

Ischaemia of the retina

Occlusion of the central retinal artery is followed some weeks later by optic atrophy (see p. 89).

Ischaemia of the optic nerve

This has two common causes – the giant cell arteritis and 'anterior' ischaemic optic neuropathy.

Giant cell arteritis. Perhaps the most important ophthalmic condition encountered in general practice, arteritic ischaemic optic neuropathy is a medical emergency. It usually occurs over the age of 60 years. There may be prodromal symptoms of temporal arteritis – malaise, weight loss, pain on chewing, scalp tenderness, discomfort when wearing a hat, and headache. Sudden and profound loss of vision occurs and a pale swollen disc is seen, with loss of direct pupillary reaction. Episodes of transient visual loss (amaurosis fugax) may have occurred previously. There is an association of cranial arteritis with polymyalgia rheumatica in about 30% of cases.

The diagnosis is all but confirmed by finding a significantly raised ESR (usually >50 mm/h) or plasma viscosity (usually >1.9). Immediate treatment with high-dose steroid by mouth is essential: the usual starting dose is prednisolone 120 mg daily, reducing as the ESR falls. The patient may be referred for a temporal artery biopsy, but treatment must come first. Failure to start adequate steroid therapy promptly may result in the even more disastrous loss of vision in the second eye. Treatment with steroids should be continued, gradually reducing the dose and finally stopping it when the ESR has returned to normal.

'Anterior' ischaemic optic neuropathy (Figure 14.3) is the cumbersome term for a condition that affects the optic nerve head and is not accompanied by giant cell arteritis. The diagnosis can only be made when arteritis has been excluded. The onset of visual loss is more gradual than in giant cell arteritis, and the loss may be less profound. The optic disc is swollen, often with associated flame-shaped haemorrhages, and there is an afferrent pupil defect. The ESR is normal.

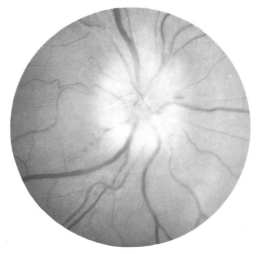

Fig. 14.3   Ischaemic optic neuropathy: note pallor of optic disc compared with Figures 14.4 and 14.6

Having excluded giant cell arteritis, other factors predisposing to arterial occlusion should be sought – hypertension, diabetes and lipid disorders. There is less likelihood of bilateral involvement in these conditions than in giant cell arteritis, but prophylactic treatment with low dose aspirin may be advised.

Optic neuritis

This is termed 'retrobulbar' neuritis if the swelling is sufficiently near the optic nerve head to cause disc swelling (see Figure 14.4). The onset usually occurs at the age of 20–45 years, but children may be affected. The cause, like that of multiple sclerosis, is not known. There is a positive association with histocompatibility antigen HLA-DR2. Certain drugs, particularly ethambutol, may cause optic neuritis.

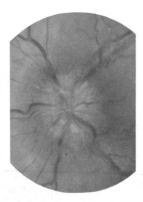

Fig. 14.4   Disc swelling: optic neuritis/papillitis: note hyperaemia, but absence of haemorrhages

The patient complains of impaired vision – perhaps as poor as mere perception of light. There is impaired colour discrimination (best shown with a red target) and a central visual field defect. The eye may be tender to the touch, with discomfort on looking to the side. The afferent pupillary defect is, in mild cases, an oscillating response to direct light. The swinging light test (p. 11) demonstrates impaired function in the affected optic nerve.

Optic nerve dysfunction can be quantified by testing visually-evoked cortical responses, and demyelination in the optic nerve can be demonstrated by MRI scanning (see Ch. 17, electrodiagnostic tests).

Treatment does not affect the outcome of optic neuritis, though ACTH or steroids may be recommended to speed recovery of vision. Most patients regain normal or near-normal vision after the first episode. More than 50% of previously healthy patients developing optic neuritis are found on follow-up to have developed other symptoms of demyelinating disease, e.g. paralytic squint (see Chapter 12), or transient blurring of vision with exercise or increase in body temperature (Uthoff's phenomenon). The exact proportion developing multiple sclerosis is uncertain. Some have no further neurological illness.

Compressive lesions of the visual pathway

These are considered below. Any patient with temporal visual field loss or unexplained loss of vision should raise suspicion of a pituitary tumour or other compressive lesion. A lateral radiograph of the skull may show an enlarged pituitary fossa. MRI scanning is the definitive investigation (Figure 14.5).

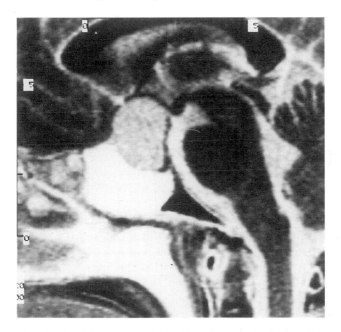

Fig. 14.5   Sagittal MRI scan of pituitary fossa: showing adenoma causing chiasmal compression

Toxic or nutritional optic nerve damage

Those most as risk from this condition are older people who smoke (particularly pipes), drink heavily and eat poorly.

Presentation is with gradually decreasing visual acuity. Defective colour perception and a characteristic central visual field defect can be demonstrated. Both eyes are affected.

Treatment is by stopping smoking, withdrawing alcohol, and giving multivitamins by mouth and hydroxocobalamin (Neo-Cytamen®) by injection: 1 mg daily for a week, weekly for a month and 3-monthly thereafter. The response to treatment is good.

Other causes of acquired optic atrophy

Glaucoma is considered on page 150, and retinitis pigmentosa on page 107.

Intrinsic tumours of the optic nerve

These rare primary tumours are of two types:

Optic nerve glioma

This is a low-grade astrocytoma, typically presenting in childhood. The tumour may spread into the chiasm and affect vision in the other eye. 15% of patients with neurofibromatosis have optic nerve glioma. CT scanning shows the fusiform swelling of the nerve.

Optic nerve meningioma

This is a rare, slow-growing tumour usually seen in middle-aged women. Presentation is usually with gradually progressive proptosis. Shunt vessels may be visible on the optic disc. CT scanning shows linear expansion and calcification of the optic nerve.

Papilloedema

Swelling of the optic disc may be due to papilloedema (Figure 14.6) or pseuopapilloedema. The distinction may not be easy.

The signs of papilloedema are:

Disc swelling
Haemorrhages near disc
Lack of pulsation of central retinal vein
Dilatation of retinal veins
Central visual acuity usually preserved.

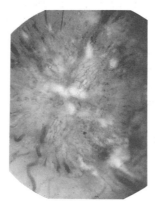

Fig. 14.6   Disc swelling: papilloedema due to raised intracranial pressure: note extensive haemorrhages and 'cotton wool' spots

Papilloedema is produced by a hold-up of the normal movement of axoplasm along the retinal nerve fibres into the optic nerve, leading to its accumulation at the optic disc. Among the causes are:

- Raised intracranial pressure, usually with headaches, worse in the morning, and on straining. Vomiting and neurological localizing signs may occur.
- Ischaemic optic neuropathy (p. 160).
- Accelerated hypertension (p. 89).
- Optic neuritis (p. 162).

Pseudopapilloedema refers to an optic disc which looks raised, but in which there is no obstruction to axoplasmic flow. The nerve fibres are functioning normally. The condition is seen in marked hyperopia and, less often, when there are drusen within the optic nerve head (Figure 14.2).

The distinction between true papilloedema and pseudopapilloedema is important, and any case of doubt should be referred. Fluorescein angiography (p. 184) may be helpful in diagnosis.

Interference with the visual pathway

The eye may serve as a guide to the presence and location of intracranial disease by the finding of visual field changes (see

Figure 14.7): rough testing can be carried out by the confrontation method. Although the lesions producing visual field defects are multiple, the types of visual loss that they cause are characteristic.

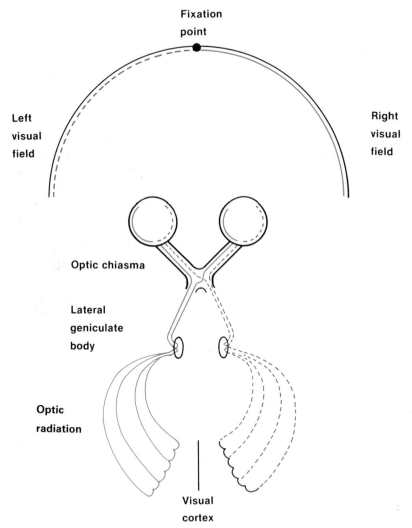

Fig. 14.7   The visual pathway

If the lesion is in front of the optic chiasm, the defect is strictly uniocular, with an afferent pupillary defect demonstrable by the swinging light test (p. 11). The optic disc is pale and atrophic.

Lesions at the optic chiasm produce bitemporal hemianopia, due to interference with the crossing fibres which carry impulses from the nasal half of each retina. This condition is typical of pituitary tumours, and the loss of field is usually asymmetrical. Impaired colour recognition is an early sign.

Behind the chiasm, any interference with the visual pathway will affect both eyes. The right optic tract, optic radiation and visual cortex receive impulses from the right halves of both retinae and damage here causes impairment of the left visual field. Similarly, the right visual field is served by the left visual pathway. A lesion behind the chiasm, therefore, leads to a homonymous field defect, lying in the same half of the field of vision of both eyes.

Running through the brain, with a synapse in the lateral geniculate nucleus, the fibres of the visual pathway terminate in the visual cortex at the occipital pole. They follow a consistent and well-defined pattern. Knowledge of the distribution of these fibres, combined with detailed analysis of visual field defects, allows accurate localization of a lesion.

Examples of typical visual field defects are given in Figure 14.8. The results of visual field analysis together with CT and MRI scans are invaluable in the investigation of intracranial disease. By far the commonest cause of homonymous field loss is a stroke involving the optic radiation. A dense defect of this type can be readily demonstrated by the GP, using the technique described on page 9.

Motor and sensory lesions

In addition to producing visual field defects, intracranial lesions may interfere with ocular movements and produce sensory changes.

Migraine (Figure 14.9)

Visual symptoms commonly precede or accompany the headache or orbital pain of migraine. Typically the patient reports a disturbance of vision which may be described as 'flashing lights'.

L   R

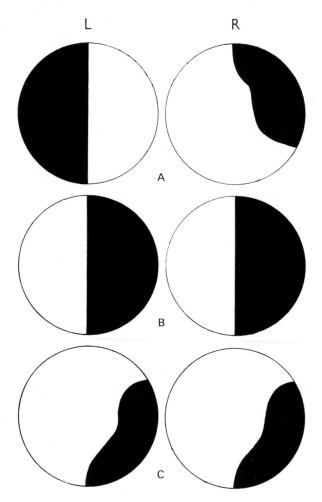

Fig. 14.8   Visual field changes, charted as seen by patient: (A): bitemporal hemianopia due to pituitary lesion – complete in the left eye, incomplete in the right; (B): homonymous hemianopia (right-sided) – complete lesion of left visual pathway; (C): incomplete homonymous hemianopa

Further questioning readily distinguishes a migrainous scintillating scotoma from the flashing lights and 'floaters' characteristic of retinal traction, due to posterior vitreous detachment and retinal tear formation.

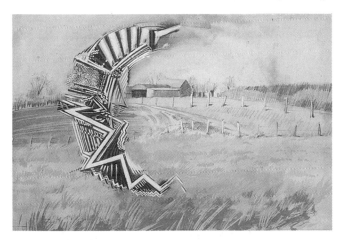

Fig. 14.9   Migraine: scintillating scotoma with shimmering spectral lights (teichopsia) (Migraine art by permission of the British Migraine Association and Boehringer Ingelheim)

Disorders of the pupil

The technique for testing pupil reactions is described on page 11.

The following are some of the commoner pupillary abnormalities:

Tonic, or Holmes-Adie, pupil. The tonic pupil is semidilated and at first seems unreactive to light. If, however, the patient is exposed to bright light for some minutes, the pupil contracts slowly and dilates equally slowly on return to the dark. This condition occurs unilaterally in young people, and is often associated with the absence of deep tendon reflexes in the lower limbs. It is not associated with serious neurological disease.

Optic (retrobulbar) neuritis (see p. 162).

Horner's syndrome. The complete Horner's syndrome comprises a small pupil, ptosis, diminished sweating on the affected side of the face and apparent enophthalmos. The condition is sometimes congenital but, if due to an active process, is caused by disease or injury affecting the sympathetic pathways.

The blind eye. In complete lesions of the optic nerve, perception of light is lost and with it the direct reaction of the pupil to light (afferent pupillary defect).

Mydriatic drugs may occasionally have been used accidentally.

Traumatic mydriasis. Direct injury to the eye may cause dilatation of the pupil (see p. 111).

Light-near dissociation. The pupil fails to react to light, but the near response persists. The causes include diabetes and disorders of the brain stem.

The Argyll-Robertson pupils of neurosyphilis are small and irregular, and react to a near stimulus while not reacting to light.

15
The orbit

Dysthyroid eye disease
Orbital cellulitis
Other disorders of the orbit
  - Orbital tumours
  - Caroticocavernous fistula
  - Trauma

Orbital disease usually presents as proptosis, the rigid walls of the orbit only allowing expansion of the contents anteriorly. Proptosis can most easily be seen when standing behind the seated patient. Measurement is carried out from the side, holding a ruler against the bony edge of the lateral wall of the orbit and estimating its distance from the apex of the cornea in profile. The two sides can be compared. Double vision and displacement of the globe are also evidence of orbital disease.

Dysthyroid eye disease

The commonest orbital problem associated with dysthyroid eye disease, proptotis, may be unilateral or bilateral (see Figure 15.1). CT scanning is indicated if the diagnosis is in doubt. Other signs of this condition are:

1. Lid retraction – the superior corneal margin is visible: under normal circumstances, the lid covers the upper third of the cornea.
2. Lid lag – the upper lid lags behind the eye in vertical movements.
3. Double vision – may result from involvement and tethering of the extraocular muscles.

The underlying cause of dysthyroid eye disease is not clear, but it may occur at any stage in the course of thyrotoxicosis and its treatment. Patients should be referred for ophthalmic assessment if complications are a cosmetic embarrassment or a risk to sight.

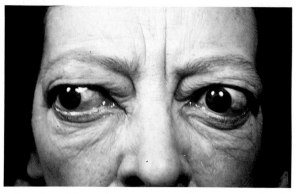

Fig. 15.1   Dysthyroid eye disease: note divergent squint due to extraocular muscle contracture and fibrosis

Hypothyroidism during the treatment of thyrotoxiocosis may exacerbate eye complications, and should be avoided.

The ophthalmic complications of dysthyroid eye disease include:

- Double vision
- Exposure keratitis (see p. 65)
- Retinal or optic nerve circulatory impairment, and secondary glaucoma.

Threat to vision may necessitate treatment with orbital radiotherapy, high doses of steroid (80–120 mg prednisolone daily) or immunosuppressive drugs; more than half the patients respond. Surgical decompression of the orbit may be required.

If the eyes fail to close properly in sleep, with risk of corneal exposure, taping the lids together at night is often helpful.

Dysthyroid eye disease is usually self-limiting. Most cases return to almost normal appearance eventually, though the condition may persist for several years, and can be independent of thyroid control.

Orbital cellulitis

Infection of the orbital contents leads to painful proptosis, difficulty opening the eye and redness of the skin. There is usually purulent discharge.

The commonest cause is sinus infection, usually ethmoiditis: confirm by X-ray examination. Skin infections, injuries, and metastatic infection may occasionally cause orbital cellulitis.

Management should be in hospital. Drainage of pus from the orbit or sinuses may be needed in addition to intensive antibiotic treatment. Preseptal cellulitis (which does not involve the eye) can be treated with systemic antibiotics on an out-patient basis.

Other disorders of the orbit

Orbital tumours

Proptosis may be due to a tumour. If the displacement is axial, the tumour is likely to be within the cone of extraocular muscles. CT scanning is of great value in diagnosis.

Caroticocavernous fistula

This causes proptosis with engorged collateral blood vessels and pulsation of the globe. An orbital bruit may be heard. Patients with this condition are invariably elderly.

Trauma

Blunt injury of the orbit may cause a 'blow-out' fracture. There is enophthalmos, limitation of gaze (usually upwards), and diplopia (see p. 115).

16
The eye in systemic diseases

Chromosomal disorders
- Down's syndrome
- Turner's syndrome

Cardiovascular disorders
- Essential hypertension
- Arteriosclerosis

Disorders of the blood
- Anaemia
- Sickle cell disease

Collagen–vascular diseases
- Rheumatoid arthritis, polyarteritis nodosa, systemic lupus erythematosus, Wegener's granulomatosis
- Giant cell arteritis (cranial arteritis)
- Behçet's disease

Other arthritides
- Ankylosing spondylitis, Reiter's syndrome
- Psoriatic arthropathy
- Juvenile rheumatoid arthritis (Still's disease)

Endocrine disorders
- Diabetes mellitus
- Parathyroid disorders
- Thyroid disorders

Gastrointestinal diseases
- Crohn's disease and ulcerative colitis

Infective diseases
- Acquired immune deficiency syndrome (AIDS)
- Tuberculosis
- Herpes simplex and herpes zoster
- Varicella
- Measles
- Maternal infections during pregnancy

Neurological disorders
- Multiple sclerosis
- Toxic optic neuropathy
- Neurofibromatosis (von Recklinghausen's disease)

Sarcoidosis

Skin disorders
- Rosacea
- Albinism
- Periocular dermatoses

The GP should be aware of the ophthalmic associations of systemic diseases, the most important of which are considered below. The information given is not exhaustive.

Chromosomal disorders

Down's syndrome

Appearance

Epicanthic folds and upward-slanting eyelids, which are shorter than normal, give a characteristic appearance in Down's syndrome. White elevated dots, Brushfield's spots, occasionally seen in the iris of normal individuals, are usually found there in Down's syndrome.

Complications

Blepharitis and trichiasis, the latter with associated corneal scarring, are frequent problems. There is an increased prevalence of keratoconus compared with normal individuals (see p. 55). This may present as acute corneal hydrops.

Cataract is common. Punctate lens opacities, which may be of little significance in early life, frequently become disabling in Down's syndrome patients as they grow older.

Children with Down's syndrome frequently develop increased refractive errors during growth and development – in contrast to normal children, who show emmetropization – a gradual elimination of the errors present in early childhood. There is also an increased incidence of concomitant squint.

Turner's syndrome

Squint is up to 10 times more common in patients with Turner's syndrome than in the rest of the population.

Cardiovascular disorders

Essential hypertension

The retinal changes associated with hypertension are described in Chapter 9. Hypertension is the principal aetiological factor in central and branch retinal vein thrombosis.

Papilloedema (p. 164) is a feature of accelerated hypertension.

Arteriosclerosis

Arteriosclerosis may cause cranial nerve palsies, particularly in the elderly, which in turn cause paralytic squints. Spontaneous recovery is usual within a few weeks (see Chapter 12).

The retinal effects of arteriosclerosis and hypertension overlap: see Chapter 9.

Transient ischaemic attacks, particularly amaurosis fugax, may be evidence of carotid disease.

Disorders of the blood

Anaemia

In pernicious and other types of anaemia, and in the leukaemias, Roth's spots – retinal haemorrhages with white centres – are seen in the fundi. They may also represent septic emboli, as in infective endocarditis.

Sickle cell disease

In sickle cell disease, peripheral retinopathy, beginning with arteriolar sclerosis and occlusions, leads to new vessel formation in a fan-like pattern. There may be sudden loss of vision due to vitreous haemorrhage, or more gradual loss due to retinal detachment. Annual retinal examinations are advised.

Collagen–vascular disease

Rheumatoid arthritis, polyarteritis nodosa, systemic lupus erythematosus, Wegener's granulomatosis

Dry eyes are a particular feature of rheumatoid arthritis. The triad of dry eyes, dry mouth and a collagen disease is known as Sjörgen's syndrome.

Peripheral corneal ulceration and/or thinning, episcleritis and scleritis may develop, and may be painful and intractable. Uveitis is not a feature of these diseases, but 'cotton wool' spots, evidence of vasculitis, may appear in the retina.

Giant cell arteritis (cranial arteritis)

'Arteritic' ischaemic optic neuropathy is discussed in Chapter 14. Central retinal artery occlusion is a rare feature of giant cell arteritis.

Behçet's disease

Recurrent, severe uveitis with hypopyon is a common feature of this disease. Treatment is difficult, and visual prognosis uncertain.

Other arthritides

Ankylosing spondylitis, Reiter's syndrome

In these conditions intermittent acute red eye, with severe iritis, is common. Patients with either condition usually show positive for HLA-B27, the frequency approaching 100% in ankylosing spondylitis.

Psoriatic arthropathy

When psoriasis is associated with arthritis, uveitis is a feature, as is the case with other sero-negative arthropathies.

Juvenile rheumatoid arthritis (Still's disease)

In the pauciarticular type (positive ANA, negative rheumatoid factor) of this condition, bilateral uveitis occurs in about 20% of patients, with insidious onset. It is commoner in females. Regular slit-lamp screening (every 4 months) is advised while the arthritis is active, usually until the mid-teens.

Cataract may develop as a complication of the uveitis; the outcome of surgical treatment is often unsatisfactory.

Endocrine disorders

Diabetes mellitus

Cataract is more common in diabetics than in normal individuals. Diabetic retinopathy and its complications are discussed in Chapter 9.

The accelerated ageing of the entire arterial tree in diabetes results in a disproportionate incidence of paralytic squint and other arteriosclerotic manifestations.

Myopia in patients with untreated diabetes, and a marked hyperopic shift when treatment is instituted, are discussed in Chapter 11.

Parathyroid disorders

Hyperparathyroidism

Calcium deposition in the conjunctiva, cornea and sclera causes red, gritty eyes.

Hypoparathyroidism

Cataracts, resulting from hypocalcaemia, are frequently seen. They usually consist of crystalline subcapsular deposits, which produce visual impairment out of proportion to their apparent density.

Thyroid disorders

Hyperthyroidism (Graves' disease)

See Chapter 15.

Hypothyroidism

Oedema of the conjunctiva and periorbital tissues may be seen in hypothyroidism. Loss of eyebrow and eyelash hair is common.

Gastrointestinal diseases

Crohn's disease and ulcerative colitis

Episcleritis and/or uveitis occur in about 10% of patients with either Crohn's disease or ulcerative colitis.

Infective diseases

Acquired immune deficiency syndrome (AIDS)

This is considered in Chapter 9. The principal sight-threatening complication is retinitis caused by cytomegalovirus.

Tuberculosis

In up to 2% of patients with tuberculosis, the infective bacteria gain access to the adnexae and the eye, particularly the choroid. Subsequently tubercles form.

Phlyctenular keratoconjunctivitis, indicating a hypersensitivity reaction, is a feature of tuberculosis. It occurs in young people with primary tuberculosis. Small, yellow nodules appear at the limbus, accompanied by leashes of vessels from the adjacent conjunctiva. Treatment is with steroid eye drops, as well as treating the underlying infection.

Uveitis occurs rarely in tuberculosis.

Herpes simplex and herpes zoster

See Chapter 6.

Varicella

Keratitis identical to that seen in herpes zoster ophthalmicus occurs very occasionally in chicken pox.

Measles

Bilateral conjunctivitis and punctate corneal ulceration occur early in the course of the disease. Generally they resolve without specific treatment. In developing countries, where nutrition is poor and vitamin A deficiency common, measles is frequently a blinding condition due to corneal damage.

Squint may be precipitated in an otherwise predisposed child of at least 2 years of age by an intercurrent illness. Foremost among such illnesses used to be measles. It has been stated, speculatively, that a decline in the incidence of squint has followed the near-elimination of measles in developed countries by routine immunization.

Maternal infections during pregnancy

The group of infections known as TORCH infections includes toxoplasmosis, rubella, cytomegalovirus and herpes simplex. Syphilis, also, is considered below.

Toxoplasmosis

See Chapter 7.

Syphilis (see also p. 170)

The triad of interstitial keratitis, malformed incisor teeth and deafness characterizes congenital syphilis. Now exceptionally rare in children, interstitial keratitis remains a significant cause of corneal opacification in older adults, who give a history of marked loss of vision for a year or two in mid-childhood, with subsequent but incomplete recovery. The slit-lamp finding of ghost vessels in the cornea is characteristic.

Uveitis of all types is a feature of both congenital and acquired syphilis, and serological testing forms part of the investigation of cases of uveitis of obscure aetiology.

Pigmented areas of the retina, alternating with areas of atrophy, give a 'salt and pepper' appearance in congenital syphilis. Active chorioretinitis may be seen in acquired secondary syphilis. Both conditions may result in optic atrophy.

Rubella

Although vaccination has dramatically reduced the incidence of rubella, 50% of maternal infections during the first trimester result in congenital infection of the embryo. The result may be microphthalmos, cataract or pigmentary retinopathy, the latter being characteristic of rubella infection. Rubella cataract may contain live virus for about 2 years, and this should be taken into account when judging the risks of surgery.

Neurological disorders

Multiple sclerosis

Optic neuritis is commonly the presenting feature (p. 162).

Nystagmus and diplopia characterize brain stem lesions. Isolated cranial nerve palsies may also cause double vision (see Chapter 12).

Toxic optic neuropathy

See p. 163.

Neurofibromatosis (von Recklinghausen's disease)

Plexiform neuroma may cause deformity of the upper eyelid. Hamartomatous lesions of the iris, Lisch nodules, are characteristic of Type 1 neurofibromatosis. Glioma of the optic nerve, causing loss of vision and proptosis, occurs in about 15% of cases.

Sarcoidosis

Young adults are principally affected by this condition. Uveitis of any type may occur, suggested by pain, photophobia and blurred vision. The slit-lamp appearance, with large 'mutton fat' keratic precipitates, is strongly suggestive of sarcoidosis. There is usually vitreous activity, with cells and other opacities. Retinal periphlebitis, with haemorrhages and sheathing of peripheral veins, contributes to visual loss.

Skin disorders

Rosacea

See Chapter 6.

Albinism

In albinism, hypoplasia of the iris, permitting transillumination, gives a pink appearance to the eye. The retina is characterized by hypoplasia of the fovea and absence of pigment from the underlying choroid. Refractive errors are common, and nystagmus is a characteristic feature.

Albinos of all types have an abnormality of the optic chiasm, as a result of which the temporal fibres from the retina decussate. Confirmation may be obtained by electrodiagnostic testing: the mis-routed decussation, in contrast to the usual hemidecussation, gives a characteristic visually-evoked cortical response (see Chapter 17).

In the ocular form of albinism, the skin may appear normal and the only apparent abnormality may be foveal hypoplasia, which is characteristic and is always present. There may be nystagmus.

Periocular dermatoses

See Chapter 3.

17
Special investigations in ophthalmology

Computerized video-keratoscopy (corneal topography)
Electrodiagnosis
Dark adaptometry
Perimetry (visual field analysis)
Provocative tests for glaucoma
Vascular imaging
   – Fluorescein angiography
   – Carotid artery imaging
Ultrasound
   – A-scan
   – B-scan
Investigation of the lacrimal system
Computerized tomography and nuclear magnetic resonance imaging

The GP will be notified of special investigations carried out and may be asked by the patient for more information about the tests and for advice about their outcome.

Computerized video-keratoscopy (corneal topography)

This is a non-contact technique involving computer analysis for evaluating the surface contours of the cornea. Topography is useful in planning refractive surgery procedures; eliminating cases unsuitable for surgery, such as those with keratoconus; and dealing with postoperative refractive problems, particularly after corneal grafting.

Electrodiagnosis

Three tests are commonly used:

1. *Electroretinogram.* The potential generated in the retina in

response to a light stimulus is detected by two electrodes, one placed on the lower eyelid and the second on the forehead. The response is diminished or abolished in widespread disorders of the retina such as retinitis pigmentosa.

2. *Electro-oculogram.* A mass electrical response is detected by electrodes placed on the skin at the inner and outer corners of the eye, when the gaze is directed to either side. The response is reduced or abolished in disorders of the retinal pigment epithelium.

3. *Visually-evoked cortical responses.* Electrodes at the occiput detect activity in the underlying visual cortex, in a manner similar to electroencephalography. A flash of light (or an alternating checker-board at which the subject gazes) produces a response, and its timing and intensity can be measured. The integrity of the pathway to the visual cortex can thus be verified in uncooperative subjects and in children. Delay in the passage of the impulse from one or both eyes indicates impaired conduction in the optic nerve – as occurs, for example, in demyelination.

Dark adaptometry

This is the assessment of the changing threshold during dark adaptation. It gives an index of rod and cone function.

Perimetry (visual field analysis)

Many devices are available for the analysis of visual fields. 'Static' perimetry involves the use of immobile stimuli of varying intensity. 'Dynamic' perimetry denotes a stimulus of constant intensity which is moved across the visual fields to determine their thresholds.

These two methods are used to detect glaucomatous field loss and other defects which may be due to neurological or retinal disease. Assessment of fitness for driving is usually by dynamic perimetry, using a bowl perimeter. Complex computer-assisted perimeters such as the Humphrey® carry out statistical analyses on the information obtained, and store it for comparison with earlier and later records. This represents a sensitive method for detecting relatively minor defects.

Provocative tests for glaucoma

Some ophthalmologists put emphasis on provocative tests in doubtful cases of glaucoma. Angle-closure glaucoma may be 'provoked' by lying the patient prone in a darkened room for 45 min (prone darkroom test), or by dilating the pupils with certain combinations of mydriatic drugs (mydriatic test), noting the intraocular pressures before and after. Patients with a tendency to glaucoma may show an increase of pressure after drinking a quantity of water (water-drinking test).

Vascular imaging

Fluorescein angiography

The circulation within the eye and in the conjunctiva can be demonstrated by photography through suitable filters after the intravenous injection of sodium fluorescein. Fundus photography displays the retinal circulation and that of the underlying choroid.

This is a particularly sensitive way of demonstrating the changes in diabetic retinopathy (p. 98). It is also of value in assessing the extent of capillary closure in retinal vein thrombosis (p. 91), and thereby predicting the likelihood of secondary thrombotic glaucoma. Prophylactic laser retinal ablation is carried out if this risk is thought to be high. Macular degenerations likely to benefit from laser treatment can be distinguished from the untreatable majority by fluorescein angiography (p. 96). This technique is also used to distinguish between true and pseudo-papilloedema, and between benign and malignant melanomata.

Intravenous fluorescein discolours the skin for a day or two and is excreted in the urine. It may cause transient nausea. In those with an allergic tendency more serious reactions, including laryngeal oedema and anaphylaxis, may occur, but very rarely.

Carotid artery imaging

Doppler studies of the carotid blood flow are useful in the investigation of transient visual loss, without the hazards of angiography using contrast media.

Ultrasound

Ultrasonic waves, generated in a probe held in contact with the eye, are reflected by the eye's structures, analysed and presented graphically on a screen. This is a non-invasive and painless technique.

A-scan

The probe is held in contact with the topically-anaesthetized cornea, and the echoes produced as the waves pass from one structure to another are measured. The most frequent use of the A-scan in ophthalmology is to determine the length of the eye prior to cataract surgery for the insertion of a lens implant. This measurement, combined with keratometry, which gives a measurement of the central corneal curvature, allows an appropriate power of implant to be calculated and is termed 'biometry'.

B-scan

This allows the eye, optic nerve and orbit to be explored in any plane. Disorders of the posterior segment of the eye can be detected in this way even when a cataract or other opacity, such as a vitreous haemorrhage, make visualization with an ophthalmoscope impossible. The technique is speedy and painless. A gel is used to establish contact between the probe and the closed eyelid.

Investigation of the lacrimal system

The simplest test of lacrimal drainage, apart from clinical examination and pressure over the sac to demonstrate retained contents, is syringing of the tear passage. Further information may be derived by radiography following injection of contrast medium into the canaliculus, or by lacrimal scintigraphy, in which a drop of short-lived radioisotope is instilled into the conjunctival sac and its passage followed by gamma-ray detector. The level and extent of obstruction are thus determined, and treatment planned accordingly.

Computerized tomography and nuclear magnetic resonance imaging

These imaging techniques are of value in demonstrating orbital and intracranial disease, complementing conventional radiography.

18
Visual standards

Screening of children for visual defects
Occupational visual standards
Visual display units

Screening of children for visual defects

The details of assessment of vision in apparently healthy children vary, but a typical screening policy is summarized in Table 18.1

Table 18.1   Screening of children for visual defects

Age	Defect sought	Type of test	Referral threshold
6 weeks	Congenital cataract Anatomical defects Squint Visual inattention – fixation – following	Red reflex	
18 months	Squint	Cover test	
3 years	Squint Visual acuity	Cover test Stycar, at 3m	3/6 or worse in either eye
School entry	Squint Visual acuity	Cover test Sheridan Gardiner, at 6m	6/9 or worse in either eye
During school every other year	Visual acuity	Snellen or screening device (e.g. Keystone® screener)	
10 years	Colour vision		

Some children of school age who are disinclined to read, and whose educational achievements are unsatisfactory, are hyperopic. The degree of hyperopia may be too small to impair distance

187

acuity, so the child passes a routine vision check, but reading is an effort. Children with reading difficulty should be referred for refraction. Most teachers and parents are nowadays aware of the possibility that a child with reading or writing difficulties may be dyslexic. Specialist advice is available from educational psychologists.

Occupational visual standards

The visual standards set for employment in the services and in industry are complex. Advice may be obtained from the following UK sources, among others:

Army, Ministry of Defence, London WC1V 6HE (or local recruiting office).
Civil Aviation Authority, Medical Dept., Aviation House, Gatwick Airport, West Sussex RH6 0YR.
Railways, Railtrack PLC and the train operating companies. Each company applies its own operating standards for operational train crew, signalmen and track maintenance staff. The general requirement is for acuities of 6/9 in the better and 6/12 in the worse eye, with glasses if worn. Drivers and potential drivers have a separate entry standard for unaided vision, of 6/12, 6/18. Normal colour vision, assessed by the Ishihara test, is required for operational staff including drivers, guards and signalmen. Information may be obtained from Operational Healthcare (Railways) Ltd., Walgate House, 25 Church Road, Basingstoke RG21 7QQ or The Specialist in Occupational Medicine, Room 23, Wyvern House, Railway Terrace, Derby DE1 2RY.
Dept. of Transport, DVLA Medical Unit, Swansea SA99 1TU. Telephone: 01792 772151.
Merchant Navy, Chamber of Shipping, Carthusian Court, 12 Carthusian Street, London EC1M 6EB.
RAF, Ministry of Defence (RAF) London WC1V 6HE.
Royal Navy, Department of General Practice, Royal Naval Hospital, Haslar, Gosport PO12 2AA (or local recruiting office).

The principal visual criterion for employment is central visual acuity, although colour vision is important in some jobs. There are variations between authorities as to whether the wearing of spectacles is permitted and, if so, of what strength.

In the UK, the required standards of visual acuity and visual fields are set by the Driver and Vehicle Licensing Agency (DVLA). The current requirements for drivers are as follows:

Car drivers

Vision is tested by reading vehicle number plates. 'Slightly better than 6/12' is the nearest Snellen equivalent to the required visual acuity. Monocular vision is no bar to holding a driving licence.

A driving licence might not be granted to a person suffering from some disability (including a disorder of the eye) which is likely to cause him/her to be a source of danger to the public when driving a vehicle. Significant loss of visual field in both eyes, e.g. homonymous hemianopia or advanced glaucoma, precludes the issue of any form of driving licence, even if satisfactory central acuity is achieved. In borderline cases a specialist opinion may be required. Patients suffering from the following conditions should notify the DVLA, so that specific inquiries about individual suitability can be made: diplopia; bilateral cataract; bilateral glaucoma; diabetic retinopathy treated by laser bilaterally; progressive retinal disorders, such as retinitis pigmentosa.

Drivers of heavy goods vehicles and public service vehicles

The required standard of visual acuity is 6/9 in the better eye and 6/12 in the worse eye, corrected. Any pathological visual field defect is a bar. A 1981 standard for uncorrected visual acuity not worse than 3/60 in either eye separately is required for new applicants.

Visual display units

Symptoms of eye-strain, as well as postural problems, are recognized difficulties which arise with the prolonged use of visual display units (VDUs). Guidelines for VDU operators have been proposed as follows:

1. The ability to read print size N6 (about that used in telephone directories) at a distance of 33–66 cm.
2. Absence of diplopia

3. Ocular muscle imbalance (-phorias) should be corrected if above specified limits:
   > 0.5 prism dioptre vertically
   > 2 prism dioptres esophoria
   > 8 prism dioptres exophoria
4. No central field defects in the dominant eye
5. Normal near point of convergence
6. Clear ocular media.

19
Blindness and partial sight

Definitions
Benefits
Useful addresses and telephone numbers

Definitions

The term 'blindness' does not necessarily imply total absence of sight. From the point of view of the social services, an individual is blind when unable to perform any work for which eyesight is essential. (Note that this definition does not mean 'unable to follow his/her previous occupation'.) In general, if visual acuity is below 3/60 the above criterion for blindness is satisfied.

There is no statutory definition of partial-sightedness, but it is a condition in which substantial and permanent handicap exists, albeit short of that justifying registration as 'blind'. Partial-sightedness usually implies visual acuity within the range 3/60–6/60, but coincident defects such as severe visual field loss may allow registration as 'blind' when the visual acuity is considerably better than 6/60.

Benefits

Registers of the blind and of the partially-sighted are maintained by local Social Services Departments in the UK. Registration is voluntary and is not usually required for services to be provided. The local Department will carry out an assessment of needs and provide information on local and national services. Rehabilitation workers are employed by Social Services Departments or by agreement with a voluntary agency to provide a range of specialist services to those with visual handicap. The aim of these services is to enable individuals to maintain their quality of life and level of participation within the community, by helping to ensure that the effects of visual impairment on daily activities are minimized. The range of specialist services provided by a rehabilitation worker includes information and advice, together with assessment and training in self-care, communication and mobility.

There follows a list of the principal benefits available to those registered as blind or partially sighted by means of Form BD8. It should be noted that some of the items listed are not available to the partially sighted, but only to the blind.

- Small reduction in cost of TV licence
- Some travel concessions
- Postal concessions on articles for the blind
- Increased Income Support and/or Disability Living Allowance
- Attendance Allowance may be available
- Income tax relief
- Special visual aids, available through hospital departments
- Advice on independent living skills and mobility
- Assessment of special educational needs
- Training in Braille and other reading methods
- Disabled parking badge
- Specialist aids and equipment to assist with all aspects of daily living
- Talking books, and tape services
- Large-print books, from local libraries
- Assessment and retraining for employment.

Useful addresses and telephone numbers

- Royal National Institute for the Blind, 224 Great Portland Street, London W1N 6AA
  Tel. 0171 388 1266
- The Partially Sighted Society, P.O. Box 322, Doncaster, S. Yorks DN1 2XA
  Tel. 01302 323132
  The Society has branches in Exeter, London, Salisbury and Wrexham. Among other functions, it takes patients by direct referral for free assessment of suitability for special visual aids.
- RNIB Talking Book Service for the Blind, Nuffield Library, Mount Pleasant, Wembley, Middlesex HA0 1RR
  Tel. 01345 626843
- British Wireless for the Blind Fund, 34 New Road, Chatham ME4 4QR (or contact through Social Services Dept.)
  Tel. 01634 832501

- British Retinitis Pigmentosa Society
  Tel. 01280 860363
- Macular Disease Society
  Tel. 01932 829311
- National Diabetic Retinopathy Network
  Tel. 0181 390 8454
- British Diabetic Association Helpline
  Tel. 0171 636 6112
- RNIB Careers Advisor
  Tel. 0171 388 1266
- Free telephone advice from DSS
  Tel. 0800 882200
- Books on cassette (Calibre)
  Tel. 01296 432339
- Newspapers on tape
  Tel. 01435 866102
- Action for Blind People
  Tel. 0171 732 8771

The above-named bodies are among the many concerned with the education, training, employment and general welfare of those with visual handicap. There are many organizations and societies which have interests in particular areas or in sufferers from particular diseases. Among these are SENSE (The National Deaf, Blind, and Rubella Association); The British Diabetic Association; The Retinitis Pigmentosa Society; Guide Dogs for the Blind; and The Disabled Living Foundation. The last-named body works to reduce the effects of disability by finding non-medical solutions to the daily living problems facing people of all ages with disabilities. Details of the addresses of these organizations, together with a summary of their aims and those of many other organizations, may be found in the 'In Touch' Handbook, available through public libraries.

Index